RECLAIM YOUR LIFE

Your Guide to Revealing Your Body's
Life-Changing Secrets for Renewed Health

DR. KARL R.O.S. JOHNSON, DC, FICPA, LCP, FIFHI

Intended Use Statement:

The content of this book is for informational purposes only. It is not meant to treat disease, diagnose, prevent, or cure any disease. The purpose of this book is to explain how using a unique blend of testing and natural treatment methods has benefited others, and how these methods can benefit you, not specifically to treat illness.

Acknowledgments and Dedication

Cover Artwork: Grateful appreciation goes out to Debra Angeline Monterosso for listening to my ideas and "Imagineering" the original watercolor for the front cover, entitled "Embrace Life," and to Kim Kavanagh for critiquing early cover designs.

Initial editing and proofing: I am indebted to Sandy Johnson, Kyle R.E.S. Johnson, Courtney L.V.V. Johnson, and Kim Kavanagh for your tireless help in editing and proofing the various chapters that make up this book. In addition I would like to acknowledge and thank Phil Thomas, Janis Clarke and Dan Cruchon for their very helpful editorial guidance.

Thanks to the multitude of patients who shared their testimonials, which add depth and meaning and real life practicality to the chapter concepts.

I dedicate this book to the millions of people who suffer with chronic illness, who have all but given up hope for their health restoration. I truly believe that the concepts and explanations in this treatise will serve you well if acted upon.

Contents

Introduction

"The doctor of the future will give no medicine but will interest patients in the care of the human frame, in diet and in the cause and prevention of the disease."

—Thomas Edison

Did you know that you will likely become addicted to prescription drugs if you have any type of chronic health challenge and live in the United States? In the spring of 2011, Dr. Oz, a noted heart surgeon, vice-chair of the Department of Surgery and Professor of Surgery at Columbia University, and host of the Emmy Award winning "The Dr. Oz Show", made the following assertions: that after seven medications, you have an 80 percent risk of drug interactions...and that *additional drugs are just treating the reactions!* As of 2004, the average number of prescription drugs taken each year, per person, was twelve, according to Greg Critser, who wrote *Generation Rx: How Prescription Drugs Are Altering American Lives, Minds, and Bodies.*

Is this where you are now, or where you are headed? Even more alarming is a recent *Los Angeles Times* report that provided this sobering statistic about prescription drugs: "Drugs exceeded motor vehicle accidents as a cause of death in 2009, killing at least 37,485 people nationwide, according to preliminary data from the U.S. Centers for Disease Control and Prevention."[1] Fueling the surge in deaths are prescription pain and anxiety drugs. Be honest with yourself, if you are not careful, you *will* be one of these statistics following the typical medical model of treatment!

Unfortunately, most of the chronic condition patients that seek my care fall into the category of those who are on many prescription drugs. Think about this incongruence: if you continue to see the same doctors, take the same medications, and practice the same eating and exercise habits, how can you expect different results? No one relishes making changes. Are you ready to live the life you *now want?* If not, my best recommendation is to throw this book in the trash; but if you are ready, read like there is no tomorrow—your life depends on it.

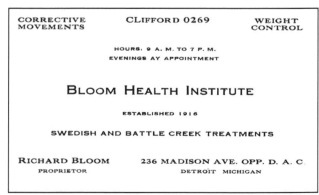

My name is Dr. Karl R.O.S. Johnson, DC. My journey into health care began with a strong desire to help people manage and heal their painful, chronic conditions. I was not the first in my family with health care ambitions. As I grew up, my mother often told stories about my grandfather, Richard Bloom, a healer from Sweden. In the 1930s and 1940s, Grandfather Bloom was a Detroit Tigers baseball trainer. Not only that, he dedicated his life to healing and to founding the Bloom Health Institute on Madison Avenue in Detroit (across the street from the Detroit Athletic Club) in 1916. He was quite a busy guy!

I never got a chance to meet my dynamic and multi-talented grandfather, but his legacy left a lasting impression on me. My mother's frequent mention of my grandfather's success with his ill clients, planted a seed that would eventually sprout into a full-blown calling to also become a healer. Like my grandfather, I wanted to help people without using the oftentimes damaging and unnecessary treatments of medication and surgery. I knew there was a vast world of understanding that I needed to explore, in order to help heal people the way I knew they deserved to be healed.

My education began at Palmer College of Chiropractic where I graduated Summa cum laude and was vice-president of Pi Tau Delta, the International Chiropractic Honor Society. As I progressed through my formal education, I was the student always asking questions. I was not one simply to take ideas, theories, or facts at face value. Rather, I strove to really understand the reasons and mechanisms behind the education I was being given. My favorite book was *Guyton's*

Physiology, which I devoured cover-to-cover, relishing the learning of how the human body works.

My first passion was chiropractic neurology, a specialized approach of looking at the brain and nervous system functionally. I was fascinated with the fact that the brain can change, remold, and create new connections when properly stimulated. The amazing ability for the brain to change is called neuroplasticity. Neuroplasticity shows us that it is possible to reveal weak areas of the brain and strengthen them through non-invasive neurological rehabilitation. Using the concepts of neuroplasticity in neurological treatment was, and continues to be, very exciting news.

I began my work by exclusively treating chronically ill patients with pain and fatigue. By using my brain-based approach, I was able to help people turn their lives around, giving them a chance to live well again after countless doctors and specialists had given up on them. In retrospect, I began to realize that when a person has a health condition that is not considered life-threatening, or if there is no easy fix for the condition, our medical system proves to be completely inadequate.

I could see the desperation in the eyes of the patients I treated day after day. They were yearning for someone to listen to them and to spend the necessary time to get to the bottom of their problem. Most importantly, they were looking for someone to help them break the chains their illness had placed around their lives.

I understood and empathized with my patients. I knew that engineering my health facility to fulfill the needs of my patients, and be the kind of doctor they needed was essential. I couldn't rush people in and out in ten minutes, and I couldn't squabble with insurance companies to pay for testing that those companies considered unnecessary. I needed to create a new way of looking at and dealing with these painful and life-changing conditions. It became quite clear that I was going to have to step outside of the current broken medical box, because inside that box was a system that could never help people in the way I knew they needed to be helped.

When using our brain-based approach, my like-minded colleagues and I were able to help many people regain their health and live free of the burden of chronic pain. However, while I was able to get amazing results with many of my patients, there were still some with whom I couldn't make the changes they needed. This subset of patients who did not respond as the others bothered me.

The most confusing part was that the patients who did not have good results seemed to have the same characteristics and test findings as the ones who were successful. I knew something was missing, and I found myself propelled on a journey to find that elusive piece of the puzzle needed to help my patients. Ultimately my journey led to the discoveries that make Johnson Chiropractic Neurology & Nutrition what it is today.

While trying to locate the missing piece, I made an important personal discovery that has forever changed my healing approach with patients. I realized that I was not looking at the body in the way most conducive to the welfare of my patients. I was doing what many doctors do, which is to compartmentalize the body, and in doing so I was missing some *very valuable* connections.

I was focusing on the brain and nervous system function without looking at the hormone system, the immune system, and the gastrointestinal system. I had an "aha" moment and I knew I would have to understand all of these systems and how they interacted with one another if I wanted greater and more consistent results. Thus began my new and continued education into the field of functional blood chemistry, functional endocrinology, and functional immunology. These combined fields of study are often termed functional medicine. Wikipedia defines this cohesive concept of healing in an accurate and fair way, "Functional medicine focuses on treating individuals who may have bodily symptoms, imbalances and dysfunctions. Functional medicine seeks to identify and address the root causes of disease, and views the body as one integrated system, not a collection of independent organs divided up by medical specialties."[2]

For a long period of time, I studied at night and on the weekends in order to further my education. I pored through scientific journals, textbooks, and articles, and traveled across the country to learn from the best teachers and mentors. I went through a period of intense research and learning, in order to become the doctor who could truly help my patients.

During this great period of study in physiology, neurology, and immunology, I made the crucial discovery that *every system in the body cross-talks with each other,* all body functions are interrelated. In order to treat and manage any chronically ill patient properly, the whole person must be evaluated; so whole-body evaluation was exactly what I began to do. Instead of only treating one part of the body, the ill part, I began to look at my patients as the intricate and extraordinary whole mechanisms they are, and made a point of running the necessary laboratory tests needed to take this big picture approach.

As I began to work using the whole-body approach, I realized most of the patients with whom I had the least success had undiagnosed thyroid problems or other undiscovered autoimmune processes. The number one cause of those thyroid problems was an autoimmune mechanism. With autoimmune mechanisms, the unruly immune system launches an attack on the thyroid gland, thus destroying it over time. Research shows that when there is one body part targeted by an autoimmune process, often the unruly immune system subsequently "goes after" other parts of the body for attack and destruction. A patient's angry immune system needs calming for patients to have hope for healing. Identifying and removing immune activating triggers, by natural means, would become an important strategy in my approach.

I applied all my knowledge about neurology, functional endocrinology, functional blood chemistry analysis, science-based nutrition, functional immunology, and body biofeedback evaluation along with natural allergy elimination, and soon I began to see big changes. I received greater and more consistent results. New patients began flying from out of state or driving from another town, after hearing from a family member or friend about their great success with us. I was and continue to be thrilled to help so many people step out of the darkness of illness and into the light of health with this in-depth treatment I call Johnson Neuro-Metabolic Therapy.

Continuous training and education is my mantra, and even after all these years, I still love learning. I have been mentored by some of America's leading functional neurologists and functional medicine specialists, and their invaluable mentoring has led me to further training through the Carrick Institute for Graduate Studies (www.CarrickInstitute. org) and the Functional Medicine University (www. FunctionalMedicineUniversity.com). I continue to learn and study functional neurology from top-notch board-certified functional neurologists in both small groups and master classes. This intense, ongoing education serves as the backbone of my ability to treat patients in a thorough and successful way.

"Dr. Johnson,

Thank you for spending the time and money to learn new ways to enhance your patients' health and well-being. Yesterday I had my first cranial adjustment. My eyesight was immediately clearer (for the past few months I had been thinking I was going to need glasses soon). My eyesight now seems to be as good as ever. But my real surprise came the next day and I'm not kidding when I say I felt 10 years younger. My energy level and stamina is like when I was 50, by the way I'm 67. Thanks Dr. J."
 - P. Tishbein, Utica

My goal in becoming a doctor of chiropractic has been to completely understand what occurs within an ill person's physiology, and then to work, *with the patient,* normalizing their bodily functions as much as possible. With normalized function, there is no need for your body to express symptoms and thus, the once noisy world of your health challenge is silenced, naturally. Writing about the concept of normal function reminds me of a quote from BJ Palmer (son of chiropractic's founder Daniel David Palmer), "Nature needs no help, just no interference".

There is a large divide between treating a set of symptoms and treating a human being. The latter requires a true understanding of what is causing the symptoms, and working on repairing the faulty physiology. The *only way* to discover the causes of the underlying problem of any health challenge is to perform specific testing.

The underlying principal and driving philosophy that guides our treatment at Johnson Chiropractic Neurology & Nutrition is that *I treat the patient, and not the diagnosis.* You are not your illness. You are a unique person with various factors contributing to your overall well-being. Each patient is treated as an individual.

Patients are never rushed into or out of my office. When you initially visit my office for a case review, I sit down with you, and go over your entire case. I formulate what advanced laboratory testing you will need, and thoroughly examine your spine, brain and nervous system from a chiropractic functional neurology perspective. After all your test results are completed, I look at your nervous system, hormone system, digestive system, immune system, and overall metabolic system to get a functional diagnosis. To obtain the best outcome, you deserve to be treated with a comprehensive, cause-driven approach.

Johnson Chiropractic Neurology & Nutrition is a premier facility for the chronically ill for a reason. I take the necessary time to make a proper functional diagnosis. Then I work with the patient to make the proper lifestyle, dietary, supplemental, structural, and neurological changes required for true healing. No other facility combines the unique healing concepts and practices like I do.

If you are suffering and need someone to get to the bottom of your condition, our center is the place for you. In this book I will discuss how I work to analyze and treat the *whole person*. I will show you how our thorough and caring process will put you onto the path of health, so that you can once again participate in and enjoy your valuable life.

CHAPTER 1

Treating The Whole Person

There is a reason most treatments for chronic conditions fail. While most doctors are looking at the disease rather than the person, they are also treating the symptoms rather than getting to the root of the illness. Patients are given medication to ease their symptoms temporarily, while beneath the medication, the underlying cause(s) of their condition worsens. This faulty method will never work to bring lasting health to the patient. In fact, it will only delay true healing. The United States' declining health statistics prove this point. The World Health Organization has carried out the first ever analysis of the world's health systems using five performance indicators to measure health systems in 191 member states. In *The world Health Report 2000– Health Systems: Improving Performance,* the U.S. health care system ranked thirty-seventh in overall performance, despite spending a higher portion of its gross domestic product than any other country.[3]

It is imperative that a person who is looking to put an end to their chronic nightmare should work with a professional who is willing to do what is necessary to unearth the cause(s) of the illness, rather than just temporarily ease it with medication. Just like anything in life that we wish to make strong, sturdy, and enduring, a solid foundation is essential. If the foundation isn't solid, then anything built on top will eventually crumble. Unless we understand and treat what lies beneath all of your symptoms, and create a new and improved structure and plan for your life, you will continue to struggle.

Most likely, you've been given a label. You've been labeled with a certain condition, and have then been given medication for it. The problem with labels is that they are generic, and they do not tell us what to do with the problem. With your unique body, genetic influences, environment, and habits, you are not generic, and neither should your treatment be generic. For example, if four people have been labeled with a thyroid problem, and each of them has been given thyroid medication, it should be no big surprise if only one of them responds well to the medication. Why does the generic approach not work? It's because there are at least twenty-four different ways thyroid physiology can go wrong, and one little generic pill is not going to fix the problem for each unique set of circumstances.

We must go deeper. You owe it to yourself to really uncover the root of your suffering. When patients come and tell me what they have been labeled, they are not giving me the information I need to help them. The problem is much more complex than many doctors would have their patients believe. A patient afflicted with a common health disorder is likely to receive appropriate care only about half of the time.[4] Only about half of the time! In other words, approximately 50 percent of people are being treated improperly.

We are trained in our society to believe that doctors know best, and when we go to a doctor, we are getting the best care. It is true that doctors are doctors because they care about people. They want to help their patients, you included. But what many patients don't understand is that doctors now function in a health care model designed to treat emergencies and simple, straightforward conditions. In many cases, doctors really just do not have the time necessary to explore your condition in a way that will actually heal it.

I am not trying to bash all doctors or medicine. I am just trying to put things into perspective. If you are a trained marathon runner, you will not be a great sprinter and vice versa. Medical doctors in the United States are groomed in medical school to treat symptoms by altering body functions with powerful pharmaceutical drugs. This one-size-fits-all mentality does not work. You would probably not be reading this book, nor be coming to my office, if it did. There is a place for medication and surgery, but more importantly, the *cause* of the problem must be identified. When this crucial step is neglected, the chance of the wrong diagnosis being given is very high. The wrong diagnosis equals the wrong care. With improper care, your frustrating chronic condition and/or pain continues to plague your life.

It is important to know that many times doctors learn about the body by studying single systems in isolation. There is a respiratory doctor, a GI doctor, a neurologist—but none of them are looking at all your systems at the same time. They are neglecting to treat you as a whole person. As a patient, you will see a handful of different doctors, and then your health issues become compartmentalized. Ultimately, the plan for your wellness is a patchwork of hasty conclusions and temporary fixes. This way will never truly work to create lasting change.

I believe that many doctors want what is best for their patients. It is the system that is broken. The pharmaceutical companies have turned human health into a business that, sadly, does not have the best interest of the individual patient in mind. The concept of a pharmaceutically hijacked medical system is a difficult truth to swallow; and one that needs to be realized and accepted if we are to turn to a new, more efficient way of understanding our conditions, getting to the bottom of their causes, and transforming them into great health.

You have to understand what is actually happening in your body to produce whatever condition is plaguing you. This understanding takes time, effort, and diligence. It also takes respect for and devotion to the process. I cannot offer you a quick fix, because quick fixes do not exist for the complex health challenges in the patients I typically see. What I can offer you is a thorough, well-rounded, individualized treatment plan. I will work hard at helping you, but you must also work hard at helping yourself. Your healing process will be a joint effort between you, your family/support system, and me!

My approach is to get to the root of the problem. I treat the whole person: your entire body, not just the ill part. I use this whole-body approach because I understand that everything in your body is working together in a dynamic and unified orchestration. It is all interrelated, each organ and gland affecting another coordinated by the nervous system. It is with this whole body approach that the body must be viewed and treated. I will order the necessary laboratory tests, perform specialized in-office testing, and evaluate every detail of these tests. After my thorough analysis, I develop your unique health recovery plan and present the plan outline to you.

But here's the catch: *you* will need to change your lifestyle. I can almost guarantee it. The first step to vibrant and lasting health is to take *responsibility* for your life. Your spouse can't do it for you, your employer can't do it for you, and I can't do it for you. Ultimately, whether or not you get well depends upon *you* and how committed you are to changing habits that do not contribute to your wellness.

Additionally, due to the specialized nature of the investigative process and treatment, most of the testing and procedures will not be covered by your insurance. Like I said before, the medical system is broken, and patients cannot rely on their insurance companies to decide which treatments and tests are truly valuable. It is important that patients seeking this treatment understand that it is not the responsibility of anyone or anything, including the insurance companies, to get them well. It is time to take it all into your own hands. It is *your life* and it is *your body* that is at stake. You must empower yourself to enjoy the vibrant life you deserve.

The great news is that the hard work pays off! You are worth the hard work it takes to have vibrant and enduring health. If you take responsibility for your life, and follow through with a *deep commitment* to carefully and purposefully transform your chronic illness into authentic health, your life will truly never be the same.

In the next couple of chapters I will explain some of the concepts behind the treatments I have found to be highly beneficial to restoring health to those with chronic health challenges, concepts that have the power to truly transform your health.

CHAPTER 2

What Is Metabolic Therapy?

etabolic Therapy is a holistic, multidimensional, big picture approach to healing and preventing illness. It is a way of shining a light on each of your complex systems, using science-based testing along with natural and highly effective solutions to heal and strengthen them. Metabolic Therapy, also known as Functional Medicine, looks deeply into the physiology of each system and into the cause of an illness, rather than just glossing over symptoms.

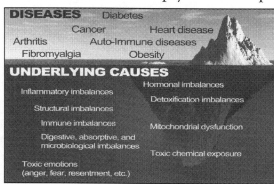

It is important to understand that in your everyday

environment, there are various factors contributing to the status of your health. Diet, nutrition, lack of exercise, and exposure to environmental toxins harm you in ways in which you are not aware. I am aware of these things, however, because it is my work and passion to know what harms you, so that I can help you. My intention is to make sure you are aware of what is keeping you from great health, and to carefully craft an individualized plan that will allow you to reclaim your life.

In practicing Functional Medicine, I am able to get to the root of each patient's condition. I am able to discover the real cause of illness, rather than just treating symptoms, only to witness their annoyingly unwelcome return. I am not interested in temporary remedies. I am interested in getting to the very bottom of what has been keeping you from great health. By handling the underlying illness factors, real change is created.

With this specialized approach, I am able to collaborate with my patients to overhaul their chronic conditions. I analyze their current way of living, so that lasting changes can be made. Once I am able to unearth the factors contributing to your illness, I can work together with you to improve your daily habits in order to bring about healing and prevent disease.

Modern doctors have *not* been trained to focus on function, which is to say that they are not trained to focus on how everything in your life is working together to create the reality of your health. Because the modern medical field has tunnel vision, doctors learn about the body in isolated systems, and focus on specific areas rather than on the body as a whole. Lacking this whole-body approach inevitably results in ineffective treatment due to the lack of crucial insight that looking at the interrelatedness of all your systems can bring.

To focus on function, it's imperative a doctor take very particular and important steps. First, the doctor must learn the physiology of each system, and how negative cycles of abnormal function become established and recurrent. In other words, he must learn the processes that are carried out by the cells, tissues, and organs, and learn where exactly these processes are not running smoothly. Secondly, the doctor has to learn what foods, nutrients, botanicals, and dietary guidelines are needed to stop these negative cycles. He must know exactly where to intervene with the proper set of therapeutic tools, in the correct order, when many of the negative cycles are working at the same time.

These things are not taught in medical school, yet they are so very important for the patient seeking *real and lasting health.* Rather than learning to understand how all of the symptoms work together, medical students are indoctrinated about how pharmaceuticals can treat the main symptoms of any given illness. Very rarely is a deep search for the underlying causes to health complaints launched. Patients do not receive thorough treatment, and they end up frustrated and in pain, or come to suffer some other form of ill health. A persona like the rebellious television physician, Dr. House, is rare indeed. And even Dr. House, with his unorthodox methods, has hardly ever used nutritional means to help his patients.

There are two schools of medicine that I would like to bring into your awareness: allopathic care and holistic care, and each carries some very critical differences. The allopathic practitioner approaches the body from the outside. He or she sees your symptoms, and prescribes medication or suggests surgery. With the allopathic approach, it is understood that everything that goes wrong with the body must be treated chemically or with surgery. The allopathic practitioner does not truly trust the body to fix itself.

Doctors who practices allopathically also do not place the necessary emphasis on the patients' roles in saving their own lives. Patients are constantly handing over their responsibility and power because they do not understand the language of their illness. Unaware of how their own bodies work, patients are ruled by fear when something goes wrong, and then they look to doctors to save them.

Fear is an understandable reaction because doctors are, after all, the people who spent years studying the human body, and are those we seek for guidance concerning our health. But the truth of the matter is that you are responsible for your own health and you must take your responsibility seriously. The days of doctors waving a magic wand are definitely over and never really existed anyway. It is only in the field of emergency medicine that our medical system shines.

As I said before, I believe that many doctors mean well. However, much of their outdated and inappropriate ways of treating patients have left many people desperate for another way of approaching health and sickness. People are beginning to sense that they will continue to hit a wall, unless they step outside of the current, broken, medical box and into a more thoughtful realm of treating their chronic illnesses.

The holistic practitioner lives and practices outside of the box. He or she sits down with patients, and takes the necessary time to listen to and understand the whole health story. This person knows that health comes from within, and trusts that the body will heal itself if there is no interference. The astute practitioner looks for factors that are interfering with the body's inborn capacity to heal, then goes about changing those factors in a joint effort with the patient, using the many natural therapies available.

The holistic practitioner has a large array of specialized knowledge about each and every system in the body, and an awareness of how they work together. He or she makes patients aware that they are responsible for their own lives, and holds them accountable for this responsibility. Accordingly, both doctor and patient work together with the patient's body to create abundant health.

Metabolic Therapy is the cornerstone for the holistic practitioner. In my experience with patients, this way of working with the body and giving patients back their power and responsibility has proven to be both empowering and transformative. Yes, I have spent years studying the human body, and yes, of course I have more knowledge about the intricate human systems than most of my patients. But I also understand the paramount importance of a patient's full engagement and devotion to their own healing. I cannot do the healing for you, and I cannot help your body to heal without you doing your part. We must work together. I will give you the tools, but you need to pick them up and put them to work. The results can mean the difference between merely surviving and actually moving through life with enough health and well-being to thrive.

What role does your brain play in this health-restoring journey? Read on to discover the awesome truth about that special organ between your ears.

CHAPTER 3

What Is Johnson Brain-Based Therapy?

Your brain is composed of many parts. There is the cerebellum in the back of the brain, and the frontal lobes located behind your forehead. Between those two parts, are the parietal 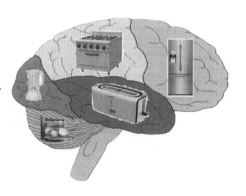 lobes, an occipital lobe, and a temporal lobe working on either side of the brain. Of course there are additional parts to the brain, but I don't want to over-complicate this discussion. Let's think of all the different parts of your brain as appliances in your kitchen. Just as each appliance has a very specific job to do, so do the parts of your brain.

Sometimes these appliances break down. If you open up your refrigerator and find that your milk has spoiled and that your ice cream has melted, then you know your refrigerator needs some tending. Similarly, when a part of the brain malfunctions, whatever is controlled by that part of the brain malfunctions too. You may begin to notice that you have severe headaches or problems with balance, vision changes, or trouble getting your words out while speaking to someone. If you are unaware of what part of the brain controls these abilities, you will not know where the weak link in your brain is located, or know what to do about it.

Johnson Brain-Based Therapy is a series of natural procedures used to identify, exercise, and strengthen weak parts of the brain by using sensory stimulation. The therapy begins with a functional neurological examination of the brain to find out where any weak links are located. When you come to see me, there are certain things you may do or feel that let me know your brain is breaking down in particular areas. Once I know where the weakness is, I am able to use natural procedures to stimulate very specific areas of your brain in order to restore function.

The human brain can be damaged, just like the skin of our bodies can. If you get a scrape on your arm, it is called a lesion. The brain can also get lesions. When brain lesions occur, it is because an area of tissue has been damaged through disease or injury. There are many types of brain lesions, some relatively harmless and some very dangerous.

There are soft lesions and there are hard lesions. Typically, hard brain lesions are cared for medically. When you have a hard lesion, such as a stroke, you obviously know you have a problem, and have probably consulted a medical doctor for evaluation and treatment. Soft or functional lesions occur when the brain is not receiving enough stimulation and, in turn, is not getting enough activity.

Soft lesions cannot be visualized with typical imaging methods such as an MRI or a CAT Scan. A functional assessment must be used to evaluate a soft lesion; I call this type of assessment a functional neurological examination. Think of it this way: take a photograph of a fully functioning, partially open door in your home. Next take a picture of a door that sticks when you close it, but photograph it in the partially opened position, as you did with the normally operating door. Now look at the pictures. You cannot tell them apart. You would have to put each door through all its actions (opening, closing, locking, etc.) while video recording the activity, for the testing to qualify as a functional test for the doors. An MRI of a brain that has a soft lesion looks normal because the MRI is not a functional test.

We must exercise our brains, just like we need to exercise our bodies, or our brains will deteriorate. Brain-Based Therapy seeks to reverse these soft lesions through stimulating your senses and training your brain to be active and healthy again. The ability for the brain to change, by adding new connections, is called neuroplasticity.

Let's take a moment to understand the great importance of your central nervous system. The central nervous system is composed of your brain and spinal cord, and it is the *master control center* and information distribution system of your body. Your entire nervous system needs both fuel and activity (stimulation) to survive, thrive, and recover from damage. Sometimes your nervous system does not get an adequate dose of these two very important elements, and that is when degeneration begins to occur.

Johnson Brain-Based Therapy takes into account that the nervous system is a sensory driven system. Each one of your senses inputs a stimulus to your brain. Your brain receives signals from your senses, and responds based on the information it receives. Without input, there will be no output. Without stimulation, the brain loses its ability to control important functions resulting in many of the symptoms of chronic illnesses.

The brain depends upon crucial sensory input to maintain healthy functioning. That is why Johnson Brain-Based Therapy is so important and effective when areas of the brain have deteriorated into an imbalanced state. I utilize sight, sound, touch, movement, vibration, heat, cold, light, and other natural tools to interrupt abnormal patterns within your brain and bring them back into balance. By using Johnson Brain-Based Therapy, I am able to strengthen the brain and effectively restore its many pathways and connections.

I have specialized tests to measure if you are receiving enough fuel and stimulation to your central nervous system. If you are not receiving an adequate amount of activation, I am able to improve the health of your brain by using specific exercises and stimulations that target weak areas. I also thoroughly check your body chemistry with lab tests for any factors that would interfere with good fuel delivery to your central nervous system. After my evaluations are complete, you and I can begin correcting these factors that impair your nervous system.

I call the combination of Johnson Brain-Based Therapy and functional metabolic testing and treatment "Johnson Neuro-Metabolic Therapy" (JNMT). JNMT is what allows me to help you when other medical practitioners have given up or failed to dig deep enough to get to the root of your chronic nightmare. There is hope using the specific rehabilitation therapies discussed in this book!

You can see it is possible to rekindle the flames of hope for getting your health back on track. You will need a guide. A mentor. Someone who has travelled the path of recovery using the tools I've explained. Your health puzzle may have many pieces that seem unrelated. Let me show you how those pieces fit to re-create the level of health you once enjoyed.

CHAPTER 4

Putting The Health Pieces Together

An important part of my role, as a health detective, is to help you put the pieces of your health puzzle together. I lay all of the factors of your health out on the table, and carefully look for the missing components. When certain pieces are missing from your health puzzle, you will not experience full health. When you are rushed into and out of a doctor's office and not evaluated thoroughly, you will never solve your health puzzle. The appropriate time must be taken, because bringing you back to health is a process. Chronic health issues that you have had for years require *time* and *patience* to reverse.

There are various factors that must be attended to, in order to change the direction of your health. The first step is discovering exactly what is wrong. Many times, patients are not given enough testing to know specifically why they are experiencing their illnesses. On other occasions, they are given the wrong tests, tests that are outdated or not sensitive enough, or the tests are being analyzed in the wrong way. No matter what health challenge a patient currently has, it is imperative that the doctor performs a *thorough* and *comprehensive* exam and medical history to determine the exact nature of the root cause of the patient's condition.

After a thorough neurological examination, I am able to determine which part of the nervous system is not functioning properly. Many times I find a high mesencephalic output. The mesencephalon is located at the top of the brain stem. A high output of the mesencephalon will cause an increased pulse and heart rate, the inability to sleep or a waking from fitful sleep, brain fog, urinary tract infection, increased warmth or sweating, or sensitivity to light. With our specialized testing, I can get very specific about what is not functioning properly within you.

What makes me unique is that I treat patients neurologically, metabolically, and structurally with added input via specialized biofeedback testing. I listen to you, and genuinely want to know your entire history, which gives important clues to illness causation. I leave *no stone unturned* to find the exact cause of your chronic condition. I use a very specific battery of tests that use samples of blood, urine, saliva, and stool to assess the condition and function of your internal organs and glands. Additionally, I use measurements of your information systems (acupuncture meridians and nervous system) to glean specific details of your body function. Thorough, precision testing allows me to know exactly what sort of individualized treatment you need to regain your health. A thorough investigation must be launched to solve your health puzzle, using Functional Neurology, Functional Endocrinology, Functional Immunology, Functional Structural Assessment and Functional Meridian Assessments. In the next few paragraphs, I'll briefly describe these assessments.

Functional Neurology is a way of working with your body's nervous system to bring it to a healthy level of performance. It aims to integrate all of the brain's sensory and motor activities, in order to bring about a correction of the abnormal function that leads to a variety of symptoms. Exercise and activations can be done using movement, scent, sound, light, and touch. Drugs and surgery are not involved.

Functional neurological testing is critical in finding out what is occurring within the nervous system. When one side of the brain becomes less functional, the other side will become more dominant. Unless the weak side of the brain is corrected, you will experience an increasing discrepancy over time. The brain will deteriorate further, and fall out of synchronization with itself, which is known as functional disconnection syndrome. I will test you for it when I do your neurological examination.

I must also look at Functional Endocrinology and Functional Immunology. Functional Endocrinology examines the causes of hormonal imbalances. I use very specific tests to evaluate why the imbalance is present. Then I use Functional Immunology to discover which part of the immune system is imbalanced. It is imperative that I test specific aspects of the immune system with very important blood tests and/or a special nutritional assessment, in order to get to the root of the problem.

From a structural perspective, when your joints are functioning in a sub-standard way, it's like having the hinges on a door rusty and stiff. It takes more effort to open and close a rusty hinge than a well lubricated, properly functioning one. Similarly, when any of the joints that interlock the 206 bones in your body are stiff or tight, your energy is wasted while moving them. From a neurological perspective, your joints, muscles, tendons, and ligaments all have nerves that send information to your brain about movement and position. Position and movement information provided to the brain is called proprioception. Abnormal structural function leads to a loss of proprioceptive information to the brain. As a result of this communication error, the output from the brain, back to the muscles and ligaments causes these tissues to malfunction. You feel the malfunction as pain, stiffness, loss of sure footedness, loss of strength, poor coordination and lowered energy. My structural assessment helps identify the areas of structural malfunction, so they can be addressed with the appropriate structural care.

Often overlooked in evaluation of patients is the meridian system of the body. Acupuncture meridians, also known as energy channels, have been used in health care for centuries. Acupuncture meridians are like copper traces on an electronic circuit board, running throughout the body. They are named by the life function associated with them. Measuring the energy of acupuncture points can be accomplished with electronic instruments such as the AcuGraph Digital Meridian Imaging system. Abnormal balance of energy in acupuncture meridians can cause disturbances in the body's ability to maintain health, similar to how imbalances in the nervous system energy can interfere with healing.

When my daughter, Courtney, was very young, she consistently woke up vomiting between the hours of 11:00 p.m. and 1:00 a.m. My wife and I would clean Courtney and her bed up and console our distraught daughter until she fell back to sleep. Finally we would go back to bed, wondering why Courtney was having this trouble. During the next day, Courtney would never show a sign that she had any illness of any kind. No sign of fever, nor lowered energy or telltale behavioral changes. Courtney's mysterious malady went on for a couple of weeks until I contacted a colleague who was familiar with acupuncture meridians, a specific set of energy channels in our bodies discovered centuries ago in the Orient. He explained how each meridian has a specific time it is purported to be most active. The gallbladder meridian was the most active between 11:00 p.m. and 1:00

a.m. He recommended I use a nutritional product to aid the gallbladder which I did, and that was the end of Courtney's nightly vomiting! Courtney's situation opened my eyes to the importance of including evaluation of the meridian system into my thorough examination of patients with chronic health challenges.

Many of my patients tell me that they don't understand why they still feel awful when all the tests they were given from previous doctors came back "normal." It is because the tests

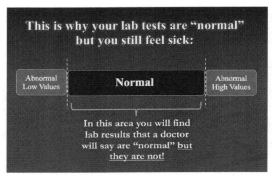

did not go deep enough, nor did the tests have tight tolerances based on optimal body physiology. At my center, I use Functional Blood Chemistry Analysis and the ranges I use are *far less forgiving*, which highlights the true discrepancies that most doctors do not discover.

Once I know what underlying causes need to be addressed and corrected, then the key factor in getting your health condition under control is *you*. You are responsible for two-thirds of your recovery, and I am responsible for

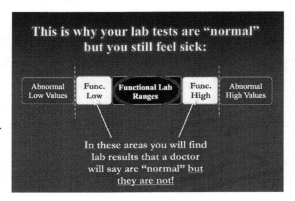

one-third. There are certain things that only you can do for yourself. I will act as a guide, offering you my education, experience, and support to steer you in the right direction, but you must work hard to stay on the path.

In order to get all the pieces of your health puzzle together, there are four aspects to Johnson Neuro-Metabolic Therapy that must addressed: diet changes, lifestyle changes, targeted nutritional supplementation and brain-based therapy. None of these aspects of care can be neglected. Those patients who are accepted into the program must be ready and willing to do what I ask of them.

The first and absolutely critical step to full and lasting health is to change your diet, based on what your tests show is necessary. There is no getting around it. We must be aware and mindful of what we feed our bodies. If your immune system has a certain imbalance, there are some foods that you can never eat again if you want to be well. On the other hand, there are certain wonderful foods and botanicals that you must eat to help you heal the imbalance. Based on your individual makeup, health-robbing food must be thrown out, while nutritious food must be embraced. Think about this analogy. How well would your gasoline engine car work if you filled the fuel tank with diesel fuel or vice versa? If you guessed that you would ruin your car's engine, you guessed correctly. People are ruining their health every day by putting the wrong type of fuel (food) in. I will help you discover the correct fuel for your unique body makeup and health challenge.

Second, you may have to get moving! Yes, I am talking about exercise. Exercise of both the brain and body are crucial to overall health and well-being. If you incorporate exercise into your daily routine, you will experience profoundly positive changes. As the old saying goes—if you don't use it, you lose it, which is actually very, very true for both your brain and your body. Other lifestyle changes may include alterations in sleep patterns and the number of times you consume nourishing food during the day. In addition, breathing exercises, meditation and/or other relaxation methods may be needed in order to bring balance back into your life.

Third, you will need to take natural supplements. Our creator made Earth full of resources that I can use to aid your health restoration. There are some very specific supplements you need to take, based on what part of your body chemistry is imbalanced. It is important that you only take what I instruct you to take. You must trust my educated judgment.

The fourth aspect of my effective health-restoring program that must be done to bring all the pieces together is Johnson Brain-Based Therapy. You will recall from the previous chapter that Johnson Brain-Based Therapy is a series of natural procedures used to identify, exercise, and strengthen weak parts of the brain by using sensory stimulation.

As you incorporate these four very necessary requirements into your life with both commitment and patience, you will begin to notice the layers of pain lifting, or your balance disorder reducing, or your numbness and tingling becoming less. By using this four-pronged approach, you and I can put an end to your chronic nightmare, and can really change the story of your life.

Another important piece of the health-solving puzzle is to detect and eliminate overt and hidden allergies, or hypersensitivities. Definitions are important and I want to clarify what an allergy is with respect to the work I employ in a treatment procedure I use to help patient's with chronic health challenges. "An allergy is a condition of unusual sensitivity of one person to one or more substances, which may be harmless to the majority of other individuals. In the allergic person, the allergic substance, known as an allergen, is viewed by the immune system as a threat to the body's well-being. For our purposes, an allergy is defined in terms of what a substance does to the energy flow in the body. When contact is made with an allergen, it causes blockages in the energy pathways called meridians, or we can say it disrupts the normal flow of energy through the body's electrical circuits. Energy blockages cause interference in communication between the brain and body via the nervous system. Blocked energy flow is the first step in a chain of events that can develop into an allergic response. Allergies are the result of energy imbalances in the body, leading to a diminished state of health in one or more organ systems".[5]

So what is this method I employ to eliminate your body's over-reaction to substances it perceives as dangerous, without drugs or shots? It's a method is called Nambudripad's

Allergy Elimination Techniques, also known as NAET. NAET uses a selective blend of energy balancing, testing and treatment procedures from acupuncture/acupressure, allopathy (the traditional medical care you've been used to receiving), chiropractic, nutritional, and kinesiological disciplines of medicine to treat imbalances that lead to allergies or hypersensitivities.[6] NAET has been found to be very effective for many acute and chronic conditions that are a result of hypersensitivity reactions. Allergies are caused by many things, including foods, drugs, vitamins, chemicals, grasses, flowers, trees, etc. In some people, contact with these substances causes severe reactions.

NAET is an energy balancing technique. It aims to enable energy flow throughout your body without restrictions. By using NAET, I am able to desensitize a patient to an allergen by applying adequate pressure directly on specific points while the person is in direct contact with the allergen being treated. The process of NAET brings about balance to the nervous system and meridian system. This process is a completely natural way of treating the patient who has allergies. For more information, please visit www.NAET.com.

Another special tool in our arsenal of testing and healing protocols is the Nano Stress Reduction Therapy (SRT) system. Think of your body's immune system as the tires on your vehicle. Certain elements on the road may cause damage to the tread on your tires, leading to misalignment, bumpy rides, skidding, and even accidents. Your tires are able to handle some elements better than others. The Nano

SRT System provides us with the data I can use to identify what elements are placing the greatest amount of stress on your body, and what adjustments, if any, may be needed to your tires (immune system) to provide the highest level of performance.

The Nano SRT system is an FDA-cleared biofeedback device and has two main components. These components have been engineered to properly assess, balance, and service the body so the immune system can maintain optimal capacity.

The first component, the Digital Conductance Meter (DCM), provide skin resistance measurements, which provides feedback necessary to properly analyze the body's energy levels. The Nano SRT provides me with your body's baseline energy measurement in addition to measurements taken when the body is exposed to various elements (stressors). Measurement parameters have been established through scientific research, to determine normal energy levels during exposure to each stressor. Any measurement readings that fall outside of these parameters may indicate a possible hazard or stress to your body, when exposed to the corresponding stressor.

Once these measurements are recorded, the second component of the Nano SRT System is used to "service the chassis." The Nano SRT Therapy utilizes the Nano SRT Focus Therapy Tool, the Nano SRT antenna, and/or a laser light wand to transmit a series of frequencies that are developed as a result of the biofeedback test, and which are unique to each individual. These frequencies are transmitted via an LED light to various meridian points on the body, acting as direct stimuli to the nervous and meridian systems. By transferring these frequencies into the body, the Nano SRT Therapy recalibrates the body's response, so that future exposure to the corresponding substances now allows the biofeedback measurements (and the body's reactions) to fall within the acceptable parameters. Your body no longer feels overburdened or stressed by the stressors.[7] For more information, visit www.ShelbyLaserHealth.com.

Over the years, I have found several ailments that, unfortunately, seem to be most prevalent in resisting amelioration. Repeatedly, patients would come to my office seeking care for these chronic conditions: fibromyalgia, balance disorders, migraines (and other debilitating headaches), thyroid disorders, and peripheral neuropathy. Using the approaches and concepts I've discussed, I am happy to say many sufferers of these debilitating conditions have found answers. Read on as I share details about how your body can reveal its life-changing secrets for renewed health for each of these conditions.

CHAPTER 5

Fibromyalgia

Fibromyalgia is a form of generalized muscular pain and fatigue that affects approximately three to six million Americans. It does not discriminate by gender or age, but predominately women between the ages of thirty-five and fifty-four suffer most frequently. The name, fibromyalgia, means pain in the muscles and the fibrous connective tissues, which refers to the ligaments and tendons.

Research has shown that fibromyalgia patients have an enhanced pain sensitivity and response, originating from central nervous system damage.[8] Traumatic illness or injury may trigger the disease. Fibromyalgia is a painful condition that lowers a person's quality of life, and leaves him or her feeling sore, depleted, and hopeless.

Pain is the most prominent symptom of fibromyalgia. Pain is generally felt throughout the entire body, though it may begin in one region and then, in time, spread to others. Most people with fibromyalgia experience moderate or severe fatigue. Lack of energy, decreased exercise endurance, and the kind of exhaustion that results from the flu or lack of sleep are common complaints. Sometimes the fatigue weighs more heavily on a person than the pain.

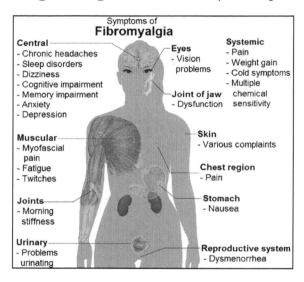

Symptoms of
Fibromyalgia

Central
- Chronic headaches
- Sleep disorders
- Dizziness
- Cognitive impairment
- Memory impairment
- Anxiety
- Depression

Muscular
- Myofascial pain
- Fatigue
- Twitches

Joints
- Morning stiffness

Urinary
- Problems urinating

Eyes
- Vision problems

Joint of jaw
- Dysfunction

Skin
- Various complaints

Chest region
- Pain

Stomach
- Nausea

Reproductive system
- Dysmenorrhea

Systemic
- Pain
- Weight gain
- Cold symptoms
- Multiple chemical sensitivity

Tension and migraine headaches are also common in patients with fibromyalgia. Other symptoms include: insomnia and other sleep disorders, depression from chronic discomfort, and multiple reoccurring infections, abdominal pain, bloating, alternating constipation as well as bladder spasms and irritability, which can cause urinary urgency or frequency. Persons with fibromyalgia find that skin and blood circulation can be sensitive to temperature changes, resulting in temporary variation in skin color.

Frequency, degree, and location of pain vary from day to day. On any given day, a fibromyalgia patient's level of discomfort may range from mild muscle stiffness to extreme pain so severe that he or she feels debilitated and unable to carry out simple activities. A common myth is that fibromyalgia does not get worse over time. Unfortunately, this notion is not the case. Studies have shown that fibromyalgia patients have greater than normal grey matter loss in the brain.[9] The longer you live with this painful condition, the worse it gets. You cannot just sit around and wait for it to go away on its own. Fibromyalgia is a functional breakdown in multiple body systems, and until someone is willing to take a step back and look at everything all at once, you are going to suffer at the hands of ineffective treatments.

Here we meet again the part of your brain called the mesencephalon, also known as the midbrain. The mesencephalon is the upper brain stem, and it acts very much like an unruly child who requires a lot of supervision. Before discussing the mesencephalon, let's first look at the neurological loop that happens in your brain.

There are two parts of your brain called the right and left cerebellum, and they are located in the back of your head. Each half of the cerebellum sends information to the opposite frontal part of your brain. The cerebellar stimulation imparted to the frontal part of your brain in turn stimulates the parts of the lower brain stem called the pons and medulla. As a result, the pons and medulla generate activity that will then decrease stimulation to the mesencephalon, thereby keeping the mesencephalon's activity in check (i.e., supervising the unruly child).

When your neurological loop is running smoothly, your brain functions the way it was designed. For example, if the right part of your cerebellum is not functioning properly, then the left front side of your brain will not get the proper stimulation, and in turn, there will be less stimulation getting to the pons and medulla. With less stimulation of the lower brainstem, the mesencephalon begins overworking, and you will experience a multitude of symptoms from this one very temperamental part of the brain.

When the mesencephalon is overworking, you can get headaches, insomnia, or pain, or you may experience light sensitivity or a racing heart. Over-firing of the mesencephalon causes increased nerve impulses, which travel down the area of the spinal cord called the inter-medio-lateral cell nucleus (IML). Increased IML activity causes the adrenal gland to release chemicals that make your pain nerves more sensitive to pain signals. The center part of the adrenal gland releases catecholamine (adrenaline and nor epinephrine) into the bloodstream. When these chemicals are released into the bloodstream, they stimulate type C pain fibers, very small nerve fibers whose job it is to transmit pain. Problems with the mesencephalon create a lot of grief. But the problems can be even more complicated, because there are many metabolic causes of fibromyalgia symptoms as well.

Diagnosing fibromyalgia is difficult. Fibromyalgia lacks laboratory abnormalities, so diagnosis of this condition depends largely upon a person's feelings and complaints. If a patient has had widespread chronic body pain for at least three months, and many different points on their body are sensitive, they will be diagnosed with fibromyalgia. Many times fibromyalgia is diagnosed through a process of elimination, and then the old prescription pad comes out to mask the symptoms of the condition.

Masking the symptoms of fibromyalgia with drugs will never solve the puzzle of fibromyalgia, and that is why many people are still held prisoner within their own bodies. The people who come into my office suffering from fibromyalgia take far more medications than any other type of patient I have seen over the years. On average, the typical fibromyalgia patient is taking eight medications!

If you only rely on medication to make you feel better, then the day is going to come when the medication simply stops working, which is fairly common. Even worse, there is no way to predict all of the awful side effects of taking that many medications, or the organ damage this overmedication could cause. Heavily medicating a patient is simply not the answer.

So how do I treat patients with fibromyalgia? I treat them neurologically, metabolically, and structurally. I strive to uncover the complicating factors that are often missed. I know that the only way to discover the causes to the underlying problem of any health challenge is to perform very *specific* testing. It is imperative that these tests are administered, so that I can help normalize patients' physiology in order to help their body restore health.

I understand that fibromyalgia is a neurological problem and an imbalance in your body chemistry and therefore, I provide the following tests and treatments:

❖ Specific neurological treatments based on specific neurological testing.

❖ Cutting edge, effective metabolic testing and specific metabolic treatment (diet, lifestyle, and nutritional supplementation), based on your specific test outcomes.

Proper testing and thorough questioning uncover the total load of stress on your body, to determine the exact cause of your fibromyalgia, and as a result, your health will have the best opportunity to improve measurably.

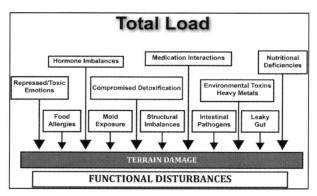

Below are detailed descriptions of some of the treatment modalities I find to be very effective:

❖ **<u>Oxygen</u>**: After about age twenty, *you lose your ability to use oxygen* by 1 percent per year! So, for example, at age forty-seven, you've lost 27 percent of your capacity. Because the ability to use oxygen goes down with age, I check oxygen levels on all of our patients. Oxygen is like gasoline in the gas tank of your car. As you get older, having enough oxygen becomes crucial. If you don't have any gas in the car, you are not going anywhere. Oxygen stimulates your nervous system to enhance healing and repair, thus decreasing pain, promoting more restful sleep, and providing many other health benefits. One focus of our recovery program is to increase your oxygen, so your brain and nervous system can do their jobs. Without oxygen available for your brain and nervous system, most likely, *no treatment will work.*

As powerful as oxygen is for healing your body, it is not enough to do the job. Fuel is not enough by itself. *Your brain must be stimulated to stay healthy, work correctly, and create healing and balance.* Below I discuss just a few of the powerful brain activations I use in my highly successful fibromyalgia recovery program to give patients suffering from fibromyalgia the relief they desperately want.

❖ **Brain-Based Therapy (BBT)** is a revolutionary breakthrough neurological treatment process pioneered by the country's leading chiropractic neurologist, Dr. Fredrick Carrick. The treatments are all neurologically based and clinically proven to help with chronic pain, balance disorders, and other neurologic conditions. The main thing you need to understand is that I stimulate the brain by using the receptors on the outside of the body that are wired and connected to the various areas of your brain. If I find weakened areas in your right parietal lobe, then I will use receptors that are neurologically "wired" to the parietal lobe, or even to areas adjacent to the parietal lobe. The process is complex, but everything I do is non-invasive, does not use drugs, and promotes proper function in the brain. The brain has an amazing ability to adapt, change, and rewire, if given the proper fuel and activation. Johnson Brain-Based Therapy is designed to promote positive neuroplasticity in your brain.

In Johnson Brain-Based Therapy I use specific tools such as:

1. **<u>Triton DTS Non-Surgical Spinal Decompression</u>**: It is exciting to be able to use the "DTS" to gently lengthen and decompress the spine, slowly stretching the muscles in the back. In turn these actions stimulate nerve receptors that activate specific areas of the brain to provide lasting relief from many of the pains from which a fibromyalgia patient suffers.

2. **<u>W.A.V.E. Pro Whole Body Vibration Device</u>**: Exercise is tough to do for a patient with fibromyalgia. Fortunately I can provide both the needed neurological stimulation and gentle exercise with the W.A.V.E. Pro®. Several research studies validating the effectiveness of Whole Body Vibration Exercise with fibromyalgia has been published.[10] By the way, W.A.V.E. stands for Whole-Body Advanced Vibration Exercise.

3. **<u>The Interactive Metronome</u>**: This computerized brain-based rehab assessment and training program has been found to be helpful with fibromyalgia and

many other chronic conditions. It combines the sound and movement stimulation to the brain that helps "rewire" brain circuits that help reduce brain fog, improve timing, coordination and concentration, as well as helping with pain reduction.

4. **Eyelights Therapy**: Eyelights were designed to provide optimal stimulation to the brain, using the optic nerve. Eyelights are glasses designed with flashing lights built to fit behind the lens, and can be programmed so I can control the intensity, frequency, and pattern of light pulses. By using specific settings, the Eyelights therapy will "wake up" the weaker side of the brain. Having one side of the brain weaker than the other is a condition I commonly find in fibromyalgia patients.

5. **ATM2**: This amazing tool is one of my favorite ones to use. Using active therapeutic movements (ATM), it provides relief from chronic neck and back pain. When your movements are painful, the brain gets used to recruiting muscles other than the intended ones to compensate for the pain. After awhile your brain memorizes the muscle activity from the painful movement, and normal pain-free movement becomes impossible. The treatment normalizes painful central nervous system controlled muscle patterns, and offers immediate reduction in pain, with long lasting results. The fibromyalgia patient goes from painful to painless in minutes, and enjoys improved and increased mobility.

6. **Cold Laser Therapy (Low Level Laser Therapy or LLLT)**: We first saw lasers in Star Trek and Star Wars. But those lasers caused bodily harm, even death to the recipient of the deadly ray of light. Cold laser therapy, however, is an FDA-cleared treatment that has been shown to decrease pain and inflammation and to speed healing, by triggering increased ATP (the energy currency of the body) in the tissues infused with specialized light frequencies. In turn, the increased ATP production speeds healing of the injured tissues. Another novel use of cold laser is to stimulate communication in our collagen[11] (the building block of all body tissues) in a way that triggers the nervous system to very quickly change muscle tone. I remember the first use of my cold laser on a fibromyalgia patient. I was pressing on a tender point and, as you might imagine, she exclaimed that it hurt. After just fifteen seconds of laser stimulation, both of us were surprised and elated to find that the tender point no longer elicited any pain when pressure was applied.

In order to unravel the metabolic mysteries of why you suffer from fibromyalgia, your body chemistry imbalances have to be assessed. I accomplish this important task via specialized metabolic testing of your systems. Some of the ones I commonly use are:

❖ **Metabolic Treatments Based on Specific Lab Panels**: Our bodies live and die at the cell level. Vibrant health relies on the ability of our system to convert the food we eat into energy. As you might imagine, the biochemical processes, collectively termed metabolism, is quite complex. Our whole digestive system is designed to break down the food we eat into absorbable raw materials for the body. All other organs and glands are involved, in one way or another, to accomplish the rest of the masterful feat of turning the raw materials into energy. To determine if the metabolic processes are functioning within health supporting tolerances, I can assess your thyroid, adrenal glands, liver, kidneys, red/white blood cells, and gut function with specific lab tests. All of those internal functioning organs can play a part in your struggle with fibromyalgia. By addressing problems with your thyroid, adrenal glands, blood chemistry, or gut function, I can help you heal much more quickly. The comprehensive tests I order include:

1. A thyroid panel of ten specific thyroid tests. When ordering blood tests, many doctors order limited panels, and as a result, many problems are missed.
2. A complete metabolic panel (CMP). The CMP allows us to check your blood glucose levels, since glucose and oxygen are needed by the brain to function properly. As a part of the CMP, I obtain tests for inflammation in your system by testing homocysteine levels, C-Reactive Protein (C-RP), and other markers such

as erythrocyte sedimentation rate (ESR), low triglycerides, fibrinogen, etc. Just about every fibromyalgia patient I have treated suffers from some form of
chronic inflammatory process.

3. A complete lipid panel that includes total cholesterol,
HDL, LDL, and triglycerides.
4. A complete blood chemistry (CBC) with auto differential. Red blood cells help me understand your oxygen carrying capacity. In addition, the immune system
function is represented in the white blood cells.

❖ **Adrenal Stress Index (ASI)**: Your adrenal glands are
your "stress" organs, meaning that they react to stress.
Being in constant pain is a stress. Most fibromyalgia
sufferers have additional emotional and chemical
stressors. If you have Stage 7 Adrenal Gland exhaustion, your blood sugar will spike and also go too low,
making your nerve cells unstable. Unstable nerves
from improperly regulated blood sugar may be one of
the reasons you have fibromyalgia. If you suffer from
insomnia, this test is very important. Insomnia is often,
in large part, due to abnormally high cortisol or abnormally low cortisol levels in the evening, when it is time
for sleep. Cortisol levels can be corrected via specific
nutritional protocols, which could end your insomnia.

❖ **Tissue Antibodies (aka Autoimmune Disorders)**: One
reason I am able to help so many patients whom others haven't is that I actively look for evidence of autoimmune disease. An autoimmune disease is where

your immune system attacks a particular area of the body. I test for specific antibodies, to determine if you suffer from an autoimmune condition. Many fibromyalgia patients that I have treated have tested positive for thyroid antibodies, and they were actually misdiagnosed. If your thyroid tissue anti-bodies (TPO and TBG) are high, you are suffering from a disease called Hashimoto's disease. The only way to find out if you have Hashimoto's is to test for thyroid tissue antibodies via blood work. If you suffer from tissue antibodies, further blood work may be ordered to evaluate immune system function, or I may have you perform an "immune quiz" at home with a specialized procedure.

❖ **H. Pylori**: Many fibromyalgia sufferers have digestive complaints as part of their myriad of symptoms. I use state of the art testing for Heliobactor Pylori (H. Pylori) bacteria. H. Pylori is a bacterium that is known to cause acid reflux, gastroesophageal reflux disease (GERD), stomach ulcers, and stomach cancer. It is estimated that about 50 percent of the world's population is infected with this bacteria.[12]

❖ **Neurotransmitters**: Neurotransmitters are vital for proper brain function. Decreased neurotransmitters can cause increased pain. Neurotransmitter imbalance can lead to the many emotional symptoms the fibromyalgia patient experiences. Neurotransmitters don't cross the blood-brain barrier; that is to say, they stay in a separated blood partition in the brain. As a result, I use questionnaires to help us understand your neurotransmitter balance. Decreased neurotransmitters can cause the increased pain, brain fog, and depression that often accompany the diagnosis of fibromyalgia.

❖ **Hormone Panels**: Symptoms related to hormone levels that are altered from what is normal may include depression, fatigue, mental fogginess, mood swings, hot flashes, sweating attacks, weight gain, and decreased physical stamina. These altered hormone symptoms are common in patients who have been diagnosed with fibromyalgia. In addition, many thyroid symptoms occur, due to the cross talk between the thyroid and the endocrine (hormone) system. Checking the saliva for unbound hormones is a very effective, accurate, and relatively low-cost way to measure hormones.

❖ **Sensitivity Testing**: Many patients with fibromyalgia and other chronic conditions have food sensitivities, or worse, an immune reaction to gluten (a peptide found in wheat, rye, barley, and their derivatives), caused by an inherited gene. I can also test you for foods that "look like" gluten to the immune system, which can also cause the same or similar reactions as gluten causes. Having these sensitivities cause the gut to be inflamed, which in turn causes brain inflammation. It is important to note that gut inflammation is characterized by bloating, not pain. The predominant symptom for brain inflammation is brain fog—just what many fibromyalgia sufferers experience regularly.

❖ **Gastrointestinal Functional Analysis**: Proper gastrointestinal (GI) function is critical to adequate nutritional status, and can impact all aspects of body function. The profiles tested address key components of proper GI health, including measurement of beneficial microbial flora (normal bacteria that live in the gut), opportunistic bacteria, yeast, and parasitic infection. The presence of abnormal disease-causing bacteria (including H. Pylori), or an imbalance of the over four hundred normal bacterial strains in the gut, can cause gut inflammation. Gut inflammation causes brain inflammation, further complicating the treatment needed to help solve your fibromyalgia. Having yeast overgrowth, parasites, fungi, or other undesirable vermin in your digestive tract can cause many of the health challenges that thyroid, fibromyalgia, and other chronic health sufferers experience, such as joint pain or brain fog. These unwanted invaders can also lead to an autoimmune attack in your body. This state of the art DNA test is supersensitive, and is often a very important piece of the diagnostic puzzle that will finally help with the resolution of your health challenge. In addition, markers of inflammation, immune function, and digestion and absorption are measured with this comprehensive test.

❖ **Increased Intestinal Permeability or "Leaky Gut" Testing**: Your intestines are supposed to allow the entry of good healthy food particles and nutrients into your body, and act as a shield to substances that are not wanted or needed, or which are damaging to the body. When your digestive tract has been damaged from inflammation or other causes, it can leak like a sieve. Conversely, your digestive tract can be so badly damaged that hardly any nourishment can come into the body, as in advanced celiac disease. I have found many fibromyalgia patients have leaky gut syndrome (LGS). LGS will also cause damage to your health due to allergy reactions, or due to immune reactions to the unwanted particles that make it into your bloodstream. LGS adds insult to injury and needs to be addressed if you are to recover your health. The only way to see if you have LGS is to test for it. So I perform this test for your health's sake.

As you can see, unraveling the reason(s) why you have fibromyalgia can be a major undertaking. Thankfully, this process of investigation can reward you with reclaiming the life you once had before fibromyalgia robbed you of your health.

Take a moment to think of your body as a house. Your nervous system is the electrical system, and your brain and spinal cord together are the main fuse box that controls everything. You can't have anything in your house working properly unless the electricity from the main fuse box travels uninterrupted over the wires (nerves). If there is a short circuit in the wiring, then nothing will work.

Just like the appliances in your house, your muscles and your vital organs need to have uninterrupted electrical signals reaching them in order to function. The electricity that your body needs to run itself is generated by your brain, and then travels to your muscles and organs through the nerves. When something blocks or alters the impulses, then your body cannot heal itself as it was designed.

Over time, your nervous system will start to break down and develop symptoms. Nervous system problems, complicated by various chemical imbalances such as thyroid malfunction, hormonal imbalances, blood sugar regulation challenges, insulin resistance, and immune system dysregulation, create a complicated set of circumstances that requires very special care.

Fibromyalgia sufferers must be treated thoroughly by professionals who are willing to handle you and your condition thoughtfully. I believe that fibromyalgia is reversible, but that it cannot be reversed with medication. You must work with someone who looks at the big picture, who observes all of your systems at once when treating this painful condition. Your recovery from fibromyalgia is dependent upon this kind of specialized care.

TESTIMONIALS

"My story begins over 15 years ago when I was diagnosed with fibromyalgia at the age of 28. My symptoms started out gradual and then worsened in a short time… In the last few weeks, I have experienced huge leaps in my health! I can go days now without ever having to nap in the middle of the day!"

"My symptoms started out gradual, and then worsened in a short time. I thought I had arthritis, and when those tests came back negative, my doctor started testing me for lupus and MS. Finally I went to a specialist who told me I had fibromyalgia. Years ago, there was not much known about this illness or the causes. My treatment for the next fourteen years centered on treating the symptoms. I spent seven years on anti-depressants, and went faithfully to a chiropractor. I lived on Tylenol when I had flare-ups, and spent many years being fatigued and in much pain. Exercise was out of the question, even though my doctor would tell me it would help. If I tried anything, even walking, I would hurt for days, and not want to get off of the couch. I would eat sweets for breakfast to give me an energy boost, because most days, I woke up feeling like I had been hit by a truck. I would continue that pattern throughout the day: craving sweets and eating them for the quick energy they provided. Being a mom of three small children, I spent my days doing the best I could to take care of them, and I always took a nap when they did, just so I could make it through the day. Very few of my friends knew what I was going through because I kept it to myself. I would put on a happy face when I was with them. When I felt really bad, I would just stay home and be extremely depressed, and not want to be around anyone, not even my family. I kept praying for a miracle. My fatigue had gotten so bad that I would get up at 7:00 a.m. to get my kids off to school, and need to take a 2–3 hour nap by noon, to be ready for them when they got home from school. Life had become a vicious cycle for me!

A year ago, I was visiting at someone's home, and heard a gal talk about her fatigue, and how this doctor had helped her. I had been praying for a new doctor that might be able to help me, so I began to ask her all kinds of questions. I was intrigued by her answers, and that her doctor used natural supplements to help her fatigue. I got Dr. Johnson's number, and made my appointment. At first, I was really skeptical of the whole idea of NAET testing. It sounded weird, and even though Dr. Johnson explained it well, I could not see how something so simple could help me. But I was desperate, and truly felt God had led him to me, so I paid for my first twelve appointments.

After my first appointment, he recommended supplements. In my mind I had made a commitment to give this a real try, so I bought everything, and began my regimen just like he said. By day three, my energy went through the roof, and I was amazed! Both my husband and I could not believe the difference, nor did I believe a supplement that my body was lacking could help like that! So my healing journey began, and it has been a great adventure. I read the book, *Say Goodbye to Illness,* and now have recommended it to my friends. I faithfully take my supplements and stick by a restricted diet, when needed, and do my home treatments! I am making an investment in my health and my future! At the end of my first year, I debated if I should continue, but when Dr. Johnson said he could get me 60 percent better, I was in! I have decided I cannot put a price tag on my health, and I don't think you should either. I have grown to trust Dr. Johnson and his wonderful staff. I call him my Miracle Man, and tell everyone who will listen about him and the results I have received!

I do want to say that in my year's journey with Dr. Johnson, I have had ups and downs. I have had weeks where I felt great, and other weeks where I didn't. I would think, at times, that this was not working, and then he would explain to me again how healing works, and that the ups and downs are part of the process. I have come to embrace that, and realize my journey to health is like peeling an onion. I go layer by layer to get to the real juicy part. In the last few weeks, I have experienced huge leaps in my health. I can go days now, without ever having to nap in the middle of the day. This winter, I skied with my husband for the first time in fifteen years, and had a blast, and no muscle achiness afterwards! I recently stood for ten hours a day for three days, at a health expo with my company, and did wonderful! Even my friend I was with was amazed at my stamina, and saw a difference from an expo I had done with her six months earlier. I have started an exercise program for the first time in years, and enjoy the benefit of increased energy, not achiness. I can take my dog for long walks again, and feel great afterwards. I don't think I truly realized how sick I was for so many years. I was in survival mode, and that is not the way to spend your life.

At forty-three, I feel the best I have felt in years! My family sees the difference in me, and so do my friends. I don't have to put on a happy face anymore, because now I wear one most every day. I am grateful to God for leading me to Dr. Johnson, and I am grateful to Dr. Johnson for his dedication to his patients and practice. Thank you, Dr. Johnson, for changing my health, and most importantly, for changing the course of my life!"

-Heather Shinsky

"I can actually say I have no pain from fibromyalgia at all."

"I saw an ad in the paper claiming there was a doctor who could help with fibromyalgia, which I was previously diagnosed with. When I first came in, I was skeptical, but in about three weeks, I noticed a lot of pain gone from my arms and all over my body. In another three weeks, much of the pain I felt in my legs was gone, and then all the pain from fibromyalgia disappeared. I can actually say I have no pain from fibromyalgia at all. I have always had dry eyes and had to wear sunglasses, sometimes even in the house. In the past two weeks, I have not had to wear sunglasses. My eyes are not dry anymore and I don't have to use Restasis like I have for the last five years. I used to wake up throughout the night from pain, and now I can sleep all night. I have had so many benefits from this program in only a short time!"

-Helen Malek, Sterling Heights, MI

"For quite a while I've suffered from fibromyalgia and hyperthyroidism... Now I can work on my feet all day in a manufacturing facility, then go home, fix dinner and still have enough energy to work in the yard..."

"For quite a while, I've suffered from fibromyalgia and hyperthyroidism. I was tired and in pain all the time. I'd go to work, come home, fix dinner, and go to bed by 8:00 p.m. My medical doctor had me on all kinds of drugs. And nothing worked.

My friend brought me to see Dr. Johnson. I come from Port Hope, two hours from Shelby, but I've had really good results.

Now I can work on my feet all day in a manufacturing facility, then go home, fix dinner and still have enough energy to work in the yard. I've been dragging logs to the fire pit and cutting grass as well as bike riding. My thyroid is coming down, too. I really feel so much better. Thanks, Dr. Johnson."

-Darla Pankow, Port Hope, Michigan

"Since I have had treatments, I have been sleeping through the night. It is incredible to be able to sleep!"

"One of the worst things about fibromyalgia was never being able to sleep. Not being able to get to sleep, and then eventually when I did get to sleep, not being able to stay asleep. Since I have had treatments, I have been sleeping through the night. It is incredible to be able to sleep!"
   - Lorraine Beavon

"I don't feel the effects from fibromyalgia anymore!"

"I've had fibromyalgia for three years, and lupus for eight years. I went to the gym for the first time in a year, and did thirty minutes, and I didn't hurt and I wasn't tired, and when I was done, I felt like I could do more. Normally I could only do ten minutes, and I would have to have a down day the next day because I would be so wiped out. I'm not tired at all now. I don't feel the effects from fibromyalgia anymore!"
   - Nicole Darr

"I haven't felt this good in twenty years!"
"I felt like I was at my wits end because I was not walking right at all and the fibromyalgia had taken over my life. The first night after my first treatment with Dr. Johnson, I slept through the entire night. I haven't felt this good in twenty years!"
   - Susan Rutherford

CHAPTER 6

Balance Disorders

A balance disorder is a disturbance that causes an individual to feel unsteady, giddy, and woozy. The person may also experience sensations such as movement, spinning, or floating. An organ in one's inner ear, the labyrinth, is an important part of the vestibular (balance) system. The labyrinth interacts with other systems in the body, such as the visual and skeletal systems, to maintain the body's position. These systems, along with the brain and nervous system, can be the source of balance problems.[13]

There are three structures in the labyrinth, known as the semicircular canals. These canals let us know when we are in a rotary (circular) motion. Other portions of the labyrinth, called the utricle and saccule, let us know if we are moving up and down, back and forth, or side to side. The semicircular canals (the superior, posterior, and horizontal), the utricle, and the saccule are all filled with fluid. The motion of the fluid tells us if we are moving. The vari-

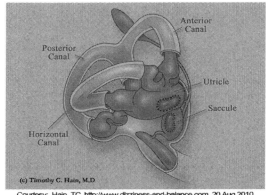

Courtesy: Hain, TC. http://www.dizziness-and-balance.com. 20 Aug 2010 <http://www.dizziness-and-balance.com/images/labyrinth-cd.jpg>

ous areas of the labyrinth, along with the visual and skeletal systems, all provide specific information to various areas in the brain that determine an individual's orientation.[14]

The vestibule is the region of the inner ear where the semicircular canals converge, close to the cochlea (the hearing organ). The vestibular system works with the visual system to keep objects in focus when the head is moving. Joint and muscle receptors are also important in maintaining balance. The brain receives, interprets, and processes the information from all of these systems that control our balance. Sometimes there is a malfunction in the way the brain receives and interprets this information, and then a balance disorder arises.

The exact number of people affected by balance disorders is difficult to quantify; in part, this is because symptoms are difficult to describe, and differences exist in the quantifying criteria within and across studies. I do know that many vestibular disorders are under-diagnosed and undertreated.[15]

Most experts regard benign paroxysmal positional vertigo (BPPV) as the most commonly diagnosed vestibular disorder. It accounts for at least 20 percent of diagnoses made by doctors specializing in dizziness and vestibular disorders. It is the most frequent cause of vertigo in the elderly.[16,17]

The most common treatment option for balance disorders is a medication, which can cause one of two things to happen. A patient may begin to feel a bit better, or not feel better at all. The medication may help as long as you are taking it, but once it wears off, the balance disorder comes back. The popular medications given for this condition cover up your balance disorder for a few hours by simply reducing your inner ear nerve's ability to send information to your brain, and by decreasing the sensitivity of your middle ear labyrinth.

Other medications are designed to destroy your vestibular hair cells, which are responsible for sending movement information from inside the utricle and saccule to the vestibular nerve. Many balance disorder sufferers do not know about the drugs they take, or that they are not 100 percent safe. In fact, many of the side effects are much worse than the balance disorder that is being treated! You can get something as minor as a rash, or you can have sudden liver failure or kidney problems. These drug side effects are scary but very real truths.

One of the most common misconceptions about balance disorders, vertigo, and dizziness is that they are solely due to inner ear problems. It is *extremely important* to understand that a balance disorder condition is not just about your inner ear or your sinuses. Chronic balance disorders are usually from a combination of neurological, hormonal, nutritional, and immune system problems. It is very complex, and the overwhelming majority of doctors and clinicians don't have any idea what to do about it.

Traditionally, treatment options for balance disorders fall into four categories: medications, physical therapy, nothing, and surgery. The medications given for balance disorders have serious side effects, and only help while patients are taking them. Physical therapists, while well-meaning, sometimes make their patients worse because they do not have a deep enough education about all the various factors contributing to the condition. When people do absolutely nothing about the condition, it is usually because nothing has worked yet, so they give up. Surgery is the most extreme option, and it is irreversible. Depending on the person, doctors may cut the nerve from the inner ear, or they may inject a drug that will destroy cells in the inner ear. Surgery is not an attractive option, especially considering that a percentage of patients receiving the surgical and drug treatment become deaf!

All of these options can be helpful to some degree, but please know that there are some very important things that they do not take into consideration. They don't ask what is causing the symptoms. They don't take into consideration the functional disconnection syndrome, which is so very critical to understanding and eliminating your balance disorder. They don't take into consideration the important parts of the brain, including the cerebellum, the parietal lobe, and the frontal lobe, which are major players in balance disorders.

Another factor these options don't take into consideration is the possibility of an autoimmune attack on your nerves, brain, thyroid, or pancreas. The common options might consider the blood sugar and insulin issue, but most likely will not. They neglect to turn the real key in treating balance disorders, and that is to determine what *metabolic* and *neurological* weaknesses exist in the individual first, and then to move forward with treatment. I have to look at the other systems in your body that may be malfunctioning and that are causing your balance problem.

Think of your brain as many different muscles brought into a cohesive whole. Some muscles can be very strong, and other muscles can be weak. When certain muscles become weak, symptoms begin to arise. I can work on these weak areas and help you to heal. If I diagnose you with a cerebellum problem, there are things I can do to rehabilitate and strengthen it.

Special consideration must be given to the cerebellum in the evaluation of any balance disorder. The four main sensory inputs to the brain that control balance and coordination come from your eyes, your inner ear, your muscles, and your joints. The cerebellum is the processing center for these inputs, in conjunction with the frontal lobe and the parieto-insular vestibular cortex (PIVC) portion of the parietal lobe. Without proper function of the cerebellum, the frontal lobe, or the PIVC, you cannot have good balance and sense of position. Since the areas of the brain need to function properly to maintain our sense of balance, my evaluation of balance disorders includes a thorough functional neurological examination of the patient's brain function.

Like any chronic patient whose symptoms last longer than six months, balance disorder patients must be monitored closely before and after treatments. If the patient is not monitored, it is possible to overstimulate or exceed metabolic capacity.

My approach is pretty straightforward. First, I ask why. What is the mechanism? Why are you having symptoms? I start from scratch, to accurately understand what is causing your balance disorder. I identify the areas of your brain that are weak, that are not functioning correctly, and then I *strengthen* them through non-drug methods, using Johnson Brain-Based Therapy.

For example, sometimes the upper part of the brain stem, that pesky mesencephalon, is firing at an abnormally high rate. If so, then I will want to utilize modalities that will lower the mesencephalic output. Then I will want to increase cerebellar output on the side and specific area of decreased output of the cerebellum.

In addition, I identify the problems and imbalances in the hormone system, GI system, and immune system, and then specifically use natural supplements along with dietary changes to balance them. There is never a one size fits all diagnosis or treatment.

So what makes my approach unique? The newest research shows that in many cases, the cause of vertigo and dizziness symptoms is an electrical imbalance in the brain, rather than a chemical one.[18] Neurological imbalance is very common in the cerebellum, the PIVC, and the frontal lobe. In scientific terms, this is called functional disconnection syndrome.

To understand functional disconnection syndrome, you have to know that there are two sides of your brain that perform very different functions. When one side of your brain becomes less functional, the other side will become more dominant. As I mentioned before, unless the weak side of the brain corrects itself, you will get a larger discrepancy over time, causing increasing problems. I am able to find out if a patient has functional disconnection syndrome by asking very specific questions and using specialized tests and tools. Hemispheric balance is very important for a healthy, functioning brain.

Think of your brain as a marching band. When both sides of the brain are working together, and they are in sync, you have a successful marching band. Everything sounds great! But what happens if the trumpets decide they are going to play half a beat off? It is not going to sound good. Similarly, when the brain is functioning in a balanced way, you get an orchestral and beautiful function. But if just one section of the brain begins to "play off tune" or "out of sync", then things get thrown out of time, and you get all sorts of symptoms like vertigo, unsteadiness, dizziness, nausea, and spinning. I need to help create hemispheric balance within your brain in order for you to be free of a balance disorder.

The newest research also shows that abnormal blood sugar levels, diabetes, resistance to insulin, and hypoglycemia all cause balance disorders. An important thing to understand is that you do not have to be diagnosed as diabetic or diagnosed with a blood sugar problem. Dysglycemia (blood sugar balance issues) is a process that can go undetected for years. You may think you don't have a blood sugar problem because all of your lab tests came back normal. But standard blood tests are faulty, due to the way in which high and low lab ranges are created.

Ranges are usually created by a bell curve analysis. The analysts gather all the results from people who have been tested at that lab location in the past year, discarding the really high results and the really low results, leaving everything in the middle to be considered "normal." Over the last twenty years, as more and more sick people have been tested, the "normal" ranges have gotten wider and wider. Overly wide lab ranges completely eliminate any real accuracy concerning your results.

In my office, I use Functional Blood Chemistry Analysis. Our ranges are much less forgiving, so I can get to the bottom of what is causing your disorder. I look at the functional disconnection syndrome, weaknesses in different areas of the brain, immune system problems, and any issues concerning blood sugar, insulin, hormones, and food intolerances. Most likely, no one has tested you with enough "breadth and depth," yet this thorough, broad-based testing is *absolutely necessary* to get to the root of the problem.

I look at these potential causes all at the same time, because if I don't, you will continue to go from doctor to doctor, losing months and even years of your life. I take the time to look at all possibilities of why you may be affected with a balance disorder, and I do it in the quickest way possible, so that your suffering may come to an end sooner rather than later.

Listed below are some of the many effective treatments that I may use to treat the cause(s) of balance disorders:

- ❖ Unilateral Adjusting
- ❖ Auditory Stimulation
- ❖ Olfactory Stimulation
- ❖ Calorics
- ❖ Unilateral Epley Maneuver
- ❖ Vibrational Therapy
- ❖ Non-Surgical Spinal Decompression Therapy
- ❖ Identifying and eliminating immune stimulating food intolerances
- ❖ Nambudripad's Allergy Elimination Techniques (NAET)

For more details about these and other treatments, please refer to *Critical Reading For What's Next* at the end of this book.

I have literally seen thousands of patients since 1983, and the one thing I can say in retrospect is that unless the underlying cause for a condition like a balance disorder is discovered and handled properly, you will only be treating the symptom. As a result, additional health challenges will crop up over time. What's worse is that these additional health challenges are usually chalked up to the "I'm getting older" excuse. This attitude is the wrong way to go about thinking about how life progresses. But when you have a dreaded balance disorder, it can be easy to fall into this erroneous way of thinking. When you seek care from a "health challenge detective," you get to the truth about your condition, and you finally can walk down the path of true healing.

TESTIMONIALS

"Vertigo and nausea gone within 2 hours after treatment…"

"I was experiencing vertigo. I was having trouble standing and functioning. My stomach was terribly upset. So I called Dr. Johnson and I came in for an appointment. He adjusted me and then he hooked me up to oxygen and at the same time that I was getting the oxygen treatment I was also doing a pedaling motion with my arms using an upper body ergometer for ten minutes. When I got done with these ten minutes, I felt immediately better after, and I felt more stable. I was able to walk out of Dr. Johnson's office and not feel any vertigo. After about two hours all the vertigo had gone from my body and I felt wonderful."

- Linda Allen

"When your body does not respond as normal, you traditionally seek a medical doctor. My story is about what happened when I followed that logic, and did not get desired results."

"For many years, I suffered from tinnitus, vertigo, and increasingly reduced coordination. I found a leading authority ENT for Tinnitus and Ménière's, and this was under control for several years. The diagnosis came out as Classic Ménière's syndrome. A no salt diet, medication, and supplements were the treatment. Tinnitus became worse, with episodes of vertigo, and then the vertigo episodes increased.

Drop attacks (severe vertigo that prevents the ability to stand) became a daily event. This situation developed over a four-year period. The symptoms became more severe, and my hearing was reduced to the point of not being able to hear from my left ear. This is the point where the discussion turned to surgical solutions involving destroying the inner ear, or cutting nerves that lead to the ear. Both solutions were not desirable for me, since I witnessed my mother suffering from the same symptoms for many years, and then have the surgery to destroy her inner ear. That was over twenty-five years ago, and following the surgery, eventually the tinnitus returned in the opposite ear, followed by vertigo attacks once again. Today she is deaf, and still suffers from these issues.

My wife was motivated to search for an alternative. Anything for relief was the task. Impacts like this start to alter your confidence, and even maintaining a conversation with someone becomes a challenge. I had to find another avenue, to provide an opportunity to beat this. Constant tinnitus, deafness, and concerns of the next vertigo attack push one to a point of frustration. I knew something was wrong, and was convinced that it was not psychological. After eating a meal, something would happen where my balance became an issue, or I suffered nausea or bloating. This was not right, and I needed to do something about it. Our search discovered Dr. Johnson and his staff. I came in for a case review, and personally discussed what was going on with me. The discussions provided an opportunity to get out from under this situation. Remember, I had been living with this, via my mother, for almost twenty-five years, and there was always a view that there was no cure.

I learned that the symptoms I was experiencing were a result of other things happening in my body. This is different for everyone. A program was developed for me, but I needed to give my commitment of time and investment for several months. I was skeptical at first, because I had never heard of a chiropractor/nutritionist resolving symptoms like the ones being experienced. I would not have believed it until one day, early in the treatment process, I had a vertigo attack with Dr. Johnson present, and he stopped the attack from accelerating. It was then that I was convinced that there is something to this.

I trusted the program, and following about six months of testing and treatments, now I have control over my balance, the tinnitus is greatly reduced, and my hearing is partially restored in the affected ear. There have been no vertigo attacks in several months, and again I have confidence to go anywhere. Following a meal, I feel energized! Again, not knowing why things happen in your body, I discovered that allergies had inflamed my body, but now I have little or no reaction when exposed to certain foods or other items.

So how did this happen? Dr. Johnson's program included determining allergies and how to eliminate them. I discovered hereditary allergies that were causing increasing issues with age, and this did require some life changes. The other allergies were eliminated through NAET. Brain-based therapy was used to rebuild my balance skills, and regular adjustments all had significant impact. The biggest impact to me was the restoration of coordination skills partially through diet changes and exercises.

The true test will be in the next six months, to determine if the great changes I am experiencing are sustainable. There will always be challenges in maintaining your health, but so far this made a dramatic positive change in my life. Thanks Chiropractic & Nutrition Wellness Center!"

-Jack F., Metropolitan Detroit

"I had been suffering from headaches, dizziness and lightheadedness for more than six months."

"When I went to the MD, he only gave me drugs, which I didn't want to take. He also told me to take Tylenol for the headaches. My friend Mary Ann goes to Dr. Johnson, and suggested I see him, and that he could help me.

My first visit was very good. Everything was explained, and the staff was quite helpful. Within a short time, my dizziness was gone. I also noticed that I had no more pressure in the back of my neck—another problem I had been having for some time. My headaches aren't so severe anymore, but I'm under a lot of stress right now, so I'm pretty tense. I'm starting the nutrition counseling this week, and with the success I've had so far, I'm looking forward to much more. Thanks, Dr. J."

-Jill Nicholas

"Allergies, ringing in the ears, sinus problems and asthma a thing of the past!"

"Here is my allergy story. I can barely remember a time when I didn't have allergies. My first reaction was to fiberglass insulation when I was about five. My father was putting in new insulation in the attic, and I decided to visit him. I soon found myself covered in softball-sized hives, and on the way to the emergency room. Penicillin was next on the list, with hives and crazy itching; no more penicillin. When I was eight, my allergies nearly killed me. Our family was in Washington, DC, for a wedding, and I had shrimp for dinner. Later that evening, I started to swell, and at one point, I couldn't see out of my eyes anymore, and my ears were sticking out like Dumbo, and the itching was unbearable. I raced to the hospital, and I honestly thought I was going to die. The doctor told my mother, who was hysterical, 'We are going to lose her if you can't calm down and tell us everything she did and ate today.' They were writing on the bed sheets, and my temperature was eighty-nine degrees. I heard my mom say shrimp, and even though I couldn't see a thing, I knew the doctors were running; after four shots of Benadryl, I was well on my way to surviving. The shots of me in the wedding pictures were another story. Those were my major allergies. As I got older, I became allergic to dogs, dust, cats, and all of your basic environmental allergies, but they were tolerable. Nearly every morning I sneezed twenty or so times, and I itched my nose so much, growing up, that I had to have nose surgery to correct the deviation.

For the most part, I could manage my allergies throughout my life, until I began a new job almost four years ago. The building was newer, but from the very first day, I smelled a strange odor in the building. As the days went by, I started noticing that my vision was getting blurry now and then. Then I started feeling off balance at work, almost like I had been drinking, and my legs would feel weak, and this strange feeling of fluid in my ears started. In the beginning, I could go home at night, and I would be relieved of my symptoms, but as the days went on, the symptoms remained with me nearly every hour of every day. I was dizzy and off-balance, my ears trickled like there was a faucet turned on inside, and sometimes I would just be overcome with nausea. I went to a doctor, and they were puzzled. She did tell me that I had fluid in my ears, and put me on a decongestant. I went back to work. My symptoms continued to get worse. I could barely function, day or night, and driving was nearly impossible, I couldn't focus at work, and my head and body felt strangely detached. I finally quit the job, after only working there for three months.

The severe symptoms did subside within a few weeks, but what remained stayed with me for years. Constantly, I had this feeling of fluid trickling in my ears, along with pressure. The really odd thing I found was that my regular allergies ceased to exist. I no longer got a runny nose or sneezed when I came in contact with an allergen. Now, all of my allergies attacked my ears, except for mold, which would revert to the old reactions, which were uncontrollable sneezing and asthma attacks. I almost welcomed the sneezing, because that I could control with medication, and when I was having a reaction to mold, the fluid feeling in my ears would stop. While Benadryl helped with the reactions to mold, it never seemed to do anything for the fluid feelings in my ears. I read many stories about how long it takes your body to recover from a sick building, and I assumed that eventually the symptoms would stop. They didn't.

Over the next year, my symptoms were annoying but manageable. My daughter and I moved into a new apartment. I checked it out thoroughly for mold and any other allergens. I was assured no animals had lived in the apartment, and it appeared clean and allergy free. I had lived in the apartment for two months when the severe allergies started again. I started getting the fluid feeling in my ears twenty-four hours a day. Then the off-balance problems started again, and I was tired all of the time. I felt intoxicated, and I was unable to focus on anything. I couldn't read because my eyes jumped all over the page. I would be overcome with sensations that felt as if I was going to pass out. My legs would feel like electrical current was running through them at night. There were constantly noises in my ears that resembled pouring milk on a bowl of Rice Krispies. I finally ended up in the hospital one day, after being overcome with these sensations.

My sister took me to emergency. I was told that, based on my symptoms, they were looking at the possibility of a brain tumor or heart problems. At this point, I didn't even care, as long as someone could tell me what in the hell was going on with me. They did a CT scan, blood work, heart monitoring, and many other tests that all returned negative. The next day, a neurologist came into see me and told me that I had Vestibular Neuronitis, also known as labyrinthitis, a non-curable vestibular condition that results in dizziness, and that I needed to make an appointment for a MRI. I remember the nurse telling me that her mother had the same symptoms, and that they never were able to help her, and that she was miserable until she finally died. Nice! I went to the neurologist for a full neurological work-up for everything from brain tumors to seizures. All test results were negative, except the neurologist told me that my eyes jumped all over, and that he noticed a large nasal polyp on my MRI, and he suggested I see an allergist.

Are you sure you want to keep reading this? So off to an ENT I go. He decides I need a CAT scan to be sure there is nothing else going on. The results come in, and he tells me I do have a polyp in my sinuses at the top of nose and in my face, and I should start with an allergist. Off to an allergist, where I have a complete work-up done, and I am told that I am allergic to everything! Not so much foods, but items like dust, cats, grasses, molds, pollens, and things that ferment. The allergist and I decide that shots are my best hope. I am concerned at this point that my apartment may have mold problems as well, since I am so sick, so my nine-year-old daughter and I move into a motel for at least a month while I look for a new place to live. I see some results from the shots and medication over the next few months. I do feel like the shots trigger a new reaction in my ear each time I get one, but overall, they are helping.

I carefully search for a new apartment, and I find one that has new carpet and paint and does not accept pets. This apartment has baseboard heat, so I don't have to worry about the dust blowing on me from the vents, which in retrospect is what was wrong with the previous apartment. An immense amount of dust came out of the hot air runs, and I was off the scale allergic to dust mites. Before I moved to my new place, I got rid of all of my plants, my curtains, and my down-filled comforters and pillows. I had to buy a new couch and mattress, because I couldn't even sit on them without feeling dizzy. I did pretty well for about a year in the new place. During this time I realized that cheese, vinegar, and alcohol were part of my allergy problem, so I eliminated those items completely. If I did eat or drink one of these items, I would feel swelling behind my nose and in my ears, and the ear sensations would last for a few days.

Last May, after dealing with this for almost three years, my severe symptoms began again, only this time much worse. I had received a promotion at work into a position that was very stressful, and I believe that was the trigger for the ensuing problems. The dizziness started in again, but this time the symptoms were slightly different. The hearing in my left ear was not very good, and I was extremely off-balance. I felt extreme pressure, bordering on pain, sometimes in that ear. My eyes were jumping around again, and this horrible brain fog would come over me. At work I could not concentrate, and there seemed to be no connection between what people were saying to me and my memory. I felt disconnected and almost drunk, much of the time. If I walked down the hallway at work, the end of the hallway would sway like I had just gotten off of a boat. There seemed to be no escaping it at home or work. I hadn't moved or changed my diet, so I was scared at what was possibly going on now.

Every few years, I would attempt to tackle this problem through medical doctors, so I made an appointment again. A very patient doctor listened to my whole story, and decided that I should see a doctor at the Michigan Ear Institute. I thought that perhaps if I got tubes in my ears, it would help with the pressure and ensuing off-balance feeling. I went to this new doctor with very high hopes. At my first visit, he did a hearing test and several other tests. He informed me that I had the symptoms of Ménière's disease, because I had low-end hearing loss, pressure in one ear, and dizziness, and my eyes were jumping around and I had the brain fog. He advised me that if I did have it, he would put me on a low salt and no caffeine diet, but he wanted to wait until the next test. This test would determine whether or not it was truly Ménière's. If you receive a positive on this test, more than likely you have it; if you receive a negative, you may still have it, but it might not be showing up.

The test was a month away.

At this point in my life, I was barely functioning, and I was deciding whether or not to go on short- or long-term disability from my job. As a single parent, I had some grave concerns about being able to take care of my twelve-year-old daughter anymore. Reading about the symptoms and prognosis for Ménière's disease left me in a state of severe depression. During this time, I started to look for alternative cures on the Internet, and started seeing a local person for cranial sacral massages. On the Internet I found that there had been some success with these types of massages, along with large amounts of B vitamins for Ménière's. I tried the vitamins for a little while, but they caused severe symptoms, and I would later find out that I was allergic to those as well. During the massages, though, there were spasms in my bad ear, which actually gave me some hope that something else was going on, other than Ménière's.

Rather than waiting for the next test and the results, I started on a low-salt and no caffeine diet. My diet consisted mostly of vegetables, rice, meat, and water. This diet was very difficult in the beginning, and I was sick for many days, especially from the caffeine elimination. But for the first time in months, I started feeling better. This was a double-edge sword for me, because I knew that if I was seeing improvement on this diet, that must mean that I must have Ménière's disease. Over the next couple of weeks, before my next appointment, I started noticing that certain foods would trigger some of the symptoms that had subsided.

Through a process of elimination, I determined that any gluten, tomatoes, oranges, and products containing MSG would send me spinning, and I quickly eliminated those options from my diet. Then the realization hit me that now, in addition to all of my environmental allergies, I had severe food allergies as well. Allergies were not curable. This was a devastating thought, but I held out some hope that if I could just manage to eat rice and vegetables, I could probably survive and be able to take care of my daughter.

My next appointment with the doctor showed that I did not have Ménière's disease, based on their tests. He did, however, say to me that the tests showed that I did not have it, but he couldn't promise me that I would not get it down the road. That was hard to hear, and I felt resentful for him putting that negative thought in my head. I discussed the food allergies, and he told me that some people that have gluten allergies do get the symptoms of Ménière's, but not true Ménière's. I decided that I should try a new allergy medicine, return to the allergist for shots, and should put a tube in my ear for the pressure. The tube did very little except bring on tremendous ringing in my ears.

This is where I found myself, and found Nambudripad's Allergy Elimination Techniques (NAET). The new job was a little less stressful, and how I made it through those months without being fired, I don't know. My diet was rice, vegetables, and meat, and I quickly lost twenty pounds, which was a blessing, but I was continuing to lose weight, and that I didn't like. The ringing in my ears was very loud at night, and I often slept with the TV on. The hearing loss was about the same. The tube fell out, and I had not returned to the doctor or the allergist. Well actually, there was one visit to a regular doctor, to talk about starting the allergy shots, but he wanted to put me on an anti-depressant first, because I don't think he fully believed me about the food allergies. I took the anti-depressants for three days, and after three days of violent headaches, I decided on no more medication and no more doctors. At work, someone had mentioned to focus on the solution and not the problem, and that got me thinking. I decided that I would find a cure for my allergies on the Internet. I found NAET and Dr. Johnson. Dr. Johnson agreed that I was allergic to nearly everything, and for the first time I was given hope, not a new prescription.

I have been in treatment for six months now, and the ringing has stopped, I am eating most foods again, the trickling feelings happen only occasionally, my hearing has returned in my left ear, and I have more good days than bad. Additionally, I rarely use my asthma inhaler anymore, unless I am exposed to mold. I still get pressure and swelling in my sinuses from my remaining allergies, and there are days where it throws me off balance and I get a slight brain fog. My allergic reactions create a very thick mucus in my sinuses that seems to change the pressure around my ear, which affects my balance. Dust is still a severe allergy for me, and hopefully I will be eliminating that soon.

I am confident that further NAET clearings will continually relieve these residual issues. The last four years have been extremely difficult, but I now consider them a blessing, because without those years, I would not have been led to find NAET treatments and the ultimate gift of having my life-long allergies eliminated.

Gratefully Yours,"

-Patrice, Royal Oak, Michigan

CHAPTER 7

Migraines And Headaches

A migraine headache is a recurrent, frequently unilateral (one-sided) headache often associated with nausea, vomiting, and sensitivity to light and noise.[19] According to the National Headache Foundation, an estimated twenty-eight million Americans suffer from migraine headaches. The World Health Organization considers this type of headache to be one of the most debilitating diseases in the world, making it extremely difficult for people to function in their daily lives.

Migraines are most prevalent in people between the ages of twenty-five and fifty-five. Women experience migraines three times as often as men, and the tendency to develop migraine headaches is often hereditary. As many as 80 percent of migraine sufferers have a family history of some type of headache disorder.[20]

Typically, the headache is a throbbing pain, much like a heartbeat. Most commonly, it is located on one side of the head and behind the eye, but many individuals have more generalized pain. Migraine is typically associated with light and sound sensitivity, nausea and vomiting, inability to do normal daily functions, and neurological symptoms of visual, shimmering lights and numbness in the body prior to the onset of the headache pain.[21]

Physical activity aggravates the pain. The pain can last anywhere from four to seventy-two hours. Occasionally, patients will have aura (visual light/neurological symptoms) without pain. These episodes typically last thirty to sixty minutes, and seem to be more common over the age of fifty.[22]

So what causes people to have these headaches? Physicians now believe that migraine headaches are caused by an abnormal regulation of pain control in the brain. The theory is that there is hypersensitivity in the neurons (brain cells) of migraine patients, and the hypersensitivity allows internal and external (environmental) irritants to trigger neurological activity in the brain, causing inflammation of blood vessels and migraine symptoms.[23]

The hypersensitive neurons may be due to a patient's genetic makeup. Common triggers of migraine headaches are hormonal fluctuations like menstruation and menopause, sleep fluctuations, neck and jaw muscle spasm, weather/barometric pressure changes, bright lights, and medication. There are also foods that excite the brain, due to added artificial chemicals like MSG, nitrates, or NutraSweet. Foods with strong smells or tastes, like aged cheese or spicy foods, can also be triggers.[24] One of the most common causes of many neurologic conditions, such as migraines, is gluten sensitivity. Often the only symptoms of gluten sensitivity and, in fact, of celiac disease, are neurological disorders, including migraines.[25]

There are five major misconceptions about headache relief. The first is that over-the-counter medications treat the cause of your migraine headache, when in fact they do not. These pills only cover up the pain by enabling your brain not to perceive your migraine headache. But the headache is still there beneath the medication, and it will come back once the medication wears off.

The second misconception is medicine can't harm you. The way these pills numb your ability to feel migraine headaches is by disabling a chemical in your body that acts like a messenger to your brain, called serotonin. Our bodies, being the highly tuned machines that they are, have figured out how to use serotonin for more jobs than one. If you disable serotonin from doing just one job, you will also disable it from doing other jobs in your body. These medications not only don't fix the underlying problem, but also cause additional problems!

Another misconception is that stress causes migraines. Stress is a part of living, but it is not the total cause of migraine headaches. It is how your body adapts to stress that determines if stress will affect your health or how you feel. I can help you increase your body's ability to adapt to stress via specific nutritional protocols.

The next huge misconception is that the recurring pattern of headaches goes away on its own. If it doesn't, you must have someone help you get to the bottom of your migraine headache, in order for the pain and chronic condition to subside.

Lastly, a common misconception is that all doctors know how to treat migraine headaches. As I have discussed previously, doctors use a one size fits all mentality that cannot possibly get to the bottom of your migraine headaches. They treat with pills, and you need treatment that goes much further than medication.

Most treatments for migraines fail for the same reasons that the treatments for other chronic conditions fail. The conditions are not thoroughly investigated, so only your symptoms are being treated. Just as with fibromyalgia and balance disorders, migraines and other debilitating headaches must be treated neurologically and metabolically.

Migraine headaches are caused by a multitude of factors. It is imperative that I understand the underlying problem first, before rushing into any treatment. Specific testing must be performed, so I am able to get further than just treating your symptoms. Finding the cause(s) and dealing with them is the only way your body can be restored so you can experience true health. I attack migraine headaches from every possible angle, giving you the best possible chance to feel like you did before the debilitating headache stole your life. The multi-pronged testing I use is a thorough and thoughtful process, and one that has the power to allow you once again to function in a healthy, productive, pain-free way.

TESTIMONIALS

"My son, Austin, suffered from migraine headaches every day."

"Two or three times a week, they would be so bad that he would throw up. He had been to an allergy MD and did shots, but they didn't work.

A friend recommended Dr. Johnson. When Dr. Johnson examined Austin, he found more than just the allergies that Austin had been treated for. Austin started NAET treatments, and soon I began to notice a difference. Austin's headaches subsided until now, when he rarely has any. Austin says that he can't remember when he had his last headache.

Austin also started receiving chiropractic care for some leg pain. Dr. Johnson said that Austin had a compressed vertebra that was causing the low back pain and the leg pain. The adjustments have really helped that too.

Thanks, Dr. Johnson, for all your help."
-Laura LaBroski, Almont, MI

"My migraines are gone and I have my energy and stamina back..."

To say that I was frustrated when I walked into your office six months ago would have been a huge understatement. Despite being young, following a very healthy diet and regularly working out for most of my life, my body seemed to be telling me I was anything but healthy. I had gone from a very active person who had completed a marathon to someone who could barely run a mile. I was lethargic, moody and constantly cold. I suffered from regular migraines, unexplained weight gain and my digestive system was a mess. I had been unsuccessfully trying to manage high cholesterol for ten years and only saw a change after finally switching to a strict vegan diet. However, the rest of my symptoms remained. I was convinced that I had a thyroid condition, even though every test my family physician ran came back normal. I was at my wits end; ready and willing to try anything in order to feel like myself again.

After you discovered that I actually had a gluten intolerance and started me on a repair and cleanse protocol, all of the pieces started to fall into place and I noticed improvement after the first week. I followed your plan religiously and could tell that my digestive tract was healing and that I was getting stronger. My energy levels improved, my moods evened out and I seem to be tolerating cold temperatures better (hopefully that holds true when winter hits!). I haven't had one single migraine since giving up gluten! I started training for another marathon and this weekend will be my last long training run - 20 miles - and I have every confidence that I will be able to complete it, and do well at the marathon in three weeks.

I am very grateful to you and to your staff for all of your help. Everyone in the office is extremely kind and supportive!

I am so happy to feel like me again!

Thank you!
-Kim C., Royal Oak, MI

"I was sure I was going blind and losing mobility..."

"Starting two and a half years ago, I began to feel symptoms where I was pretty sure I was going blind and was losing my mobility. I was beginning to kind of curl up into a little ball, into the fetal position. I am used to taking walks to the extent of three to five miles at a time. I enjoy long, fast walks. I reached a point where I couldn't walk more than a couple hundred feet without starting to weave like I was drunk. I had balance problems, extreme light sensitivity, and headaches. I couldn't keep my eyes open, and had to pry them open to drive. I stopped driving because it got so bad that I trashed my car.

I spent $12,000 on co-pays while my insurance company spent $60,000 on medical related stuff for two years, and they found nothing wrong with me.

I started BBT (Brain-Based Therapy) treatments and NAET treatments based on faith in Dr. Johnson. There's music as part of the therapy, as well as diet and supplements. It's everything working together and at the same time. I am here to tell you that it works!

I am back to walking. I took a one-mile walk yesterday, and I wasn't even concerned or scared, and I sure wasn't winded. I'm really looking forward to going on vacation to walk the beach, which I haven't done in three years.

Dr. Johnson has eliminated the headaches, so Ron is a happy camper!"

-Ron Toomer, Sterling Heights, MI

"I would like to give you a great big hug and thank-you for the wonderful care that I have always received here at the wellness center."

"When I first came to your office, I was a little skeptical about the need for chiropractic care. You hear so much from people who don't know the benefits of chiropractic care, and start to believe that you will never need it either. But I definitely did.

Before coming to the clinic, I had experienced frequent migraines and neck pain with chronic insomnia. I had missed a lot of work, and had seen many neurologists to no avail. I also received paralytics that were injected into my head to numb the right side of my head so the pain would not be so bad, so I could continue to work and support my family. I received multiple injections, and tried just about every migraine medication on the market. I was desperate for help.

I had frequent ER visits, and in one episode, I was up for five days with pain so intense I could not sleep without strong prescription sleeping medication. My body just would not sleep. A friend at my church recommended Dr. Johnson. I was hoping Dr. Johnson would find something the others had not. Dr. Johnson told me that I had heavy metal toxicity and TMJ, with subluxation to my neck.

I also forgot to mention another problem I had, which was weekly menstrual periods that were left uncorrected by progesterone from the ob-gyn. After two weeks of adjustments by Dr. Johnson, my weekly periods had stopped and had normalized! And my sleeping slowly started improving with NAET treatments and supplements. Dr. Johnson had explained that my head was in vasospasm. Because of Dr. Johnson's diagnosis, I was able to get the corrective TMJ splint that I needed to stop the continued vasospasm in my head.

I truly believe that if I had not been seen by Dr. Johnson I would still be suffering at a magnitude too much to continue working. I am so grateful to Dr. Johnson for staying in this profession. This is one of those life experiences that you are very grateful that you had experienced. And I am truly a believer in Jesus Christ, and that he causes all things to work for our good, for those that love him and are called according to his purpose. And through this experience, I have seen the goodness in others, like Dr. Johnson sacrificing their time to help others, which has been a blessing to me. And in return, I have a greater compassion through the pain I suffered, for those who are suffering too, which causes me to do more for others and go that extra mile to be a blessing to others.

In return, life is so much more rewarding now for me. I work in one of the biggest hospitals in the state, and I see a lot of suffering.

I tell many people about Dr. Johnson and the benefits that I have experienced. I tell a friend, and she tells her father in law, and so forth. I just print off their website page and hope they will get the help they need too. I truly believe that Dr. Johnson is an answer to my prayer and my family's prayers. God bless you Dr. Johnson! And I would like to sincerely say, "Thank-You!" from the bottom of my heart. I will always be thankful to you and your kind staff for all the benefits that I have experienced through your care.

You truly are a Godsend..."

-Lisa Sack, Clawson, Michigan

"For fifteen-plus years, I suffered from extremely severe migraine-like headaches."

Sometimes they were so bad that I would vomit for hours. They sapped all my energy, and often I could not function normally at all. This whole thing impacted my family, my friends, my marriage, my work, and my fun.

I had seen many doctors, and had had MRIs and lots of different tests done. I saw my family physician, allergist, ENT specialist, and a surgeon. They put me on lots of drugs, shots, antibiotics, etc.

When I had just about reached my end and was ready to try anything, my friend recommended Dr. Johnson. Dr.

Johnson and his staff were great. They were very thorough—x-rays, hand grip, foot weight, bending, etc.

Dr. Johnson told me that my problem was my neck, not my head. The adjustments started helping immediately. Then, when I added nutrition to the program, good things really began happening.

I've been with the clinic since March 1996, and I can honestly recommend Dr. Johnson's care to others. It can help restore the natural energy that is in all of us. No one should have to go through what I went through for way too many years. Dr. Johnson and his staff really care about their patients."

-B. W., Troy, MI

"For years I was my medical doctor's guinea pig."

I suffered from severe headaches, migraines, almost daily for four years after my child was born. My doctor gave me prescription after prescription for allergy pills. I got very little relief, and my allergies kept increasing.

My mom is a patient at Dr. Johnson's, and she highly recommended him to me. I've been coming for about four months now, and I'm noticing a big difference already. I haven't used any pills or nasal sprays for about three months now. I have more energy and only about one migraine every other week.

My ten-year-old daughter also suffers from allergies, and has been coming to Dr. Johnson for about three months now, and she is also doing much better with care from Dr. Johnson.

I'm happy to recommend Dr. Johnson to everyone. He's really been a great help."

-Kristine Kot, New Haven, MI

"For over five years, I've suffered from severe migraine headaches."

I went to all kinds of doctors, even neurologists. I'd have four to seven migraines each week, and found it difficult to do most anything during a headache. I took all kinds of drugs, hoping for relief, but I only felt worse, sometimes fuzzy, and the pain never totally went away.

For years, my friends who are Dr. Johnson's patients tried to get me to come to him. Finally I said, "What have I got to lose?" and made my appointment.

I started getting adjusted, and within ten days, I noticed a difference. I've only been coming for three weeks now, but I haven't had a severe headache in one and a half weeks—a record for me.

I'm really pleased with my care here, and I look forward to feeling better and better. Thanks, Dr. Johnson."

-Dianne McEwen, Macomb Twp., MI

CHAPTER 8

Thyroid Disorders

The thyroid is a small butterfly-shaped gland located in the front of the neck. It is made up of two halves, called lobes, that lie along the windpipe (trachea) and are joined together by a narrow band of thyroid tissue, known as the isthmus. Though it weighs only about an ounce, the thyroid gland has some very important functions to carry out that have a major impact on one's health. It maintains body temperature, controls the rate of energy production (including oxygen use and basal metabolic rate), regulates the skeletal and muscular growth of children, and heavily influences brain chemistry. Additionally, the thyroid gland has major influence in many other areas. The very important thyroid:

❖ Enhances a portion of the nervous system called the sympathetic nervous system (SNS).

❖ Promotes breakdown of blood sugar, and mobilizes fats essential for protein synthesis.

❖ Enhances the liver's synthesis of cholesterol.

❖ Promotes normal adult nervous system function and mood.

❖ Promotes normal functioning of the heart.

❖ Promotes normal muscular growth and function.

❖ Promotes normal GI motility and tone.

❖ Increases secretion of digestive juices, particularly those of the gall bladder and the stomach.

❖ Promotes normal female reproductive ability and lactation.

❖ Promotes normal hydration and secretory activity of the skin.

The thyroid gland takes iodine, a chemical element found in many foods, and converts it into the thyroid hormones, thyroxin (T4) and triiodothyronine (T3). It is estimated that iodine makes up about 0.00004 percent of the total human body weight, and that it is found in highest concentration in the thyroid gland cells. The thyroid gland cells combine iodine and the amino acid, tyrosine, to make the hormones, T4 (thyroxin) and T3 (triiodothyronine). These hormones are then released into the bloodstream and transported throughout the body, attached mainly to a protein called thyroxine-binding globulin (TGB). Thyroid hormones control metabolism (conversion of oxygen and calories to energy). Every cell in the body depends upon thyroid hormones for regulation of their metabolism.

It is important to understand that T4 is an inactive thyroid hormone, and that approximately 93 percent of the thyroid's production of hormone is T4. Only about 3 percent of the hormone that the thyroid gland produces is active thyroid hormone (T3), however, T3 possesses about four times the hormone "strength" as T4. The 93 percent inactive T4 hormone must be converted to T3 in order for this active hormone to generate all the important effects in the body. Reportedly, 60 percent of T4 is converted to T3 in the liver, and 20 percent is converted into another inactive thyroid hormone called reverse T3 (rT3). Another 20 percent of T4 is converted to T3 Sulfate (T3S) and triiodothyroacetic acid (T3AC) through the action of the digestive tract bacteria (assuming that your digestive tract is in a healthy balance of bacteria), and fully converted to T3. Any remaining T4 hormone that wasn't transformed into T3 or inactive T3 forms will be converted into T3 by the peripheral tissues (found in brain cells and muscle cells). Only the active T3 hormone exerts its controlling effect on metabolism and on all the other functions it governs or modulates. All this physiology sounds a bit complicated, but it is very important to learn about. For clarification, take a look at the diagram on the next page that shows all these steps and processes it takes to make thyroid hormones active in the body.

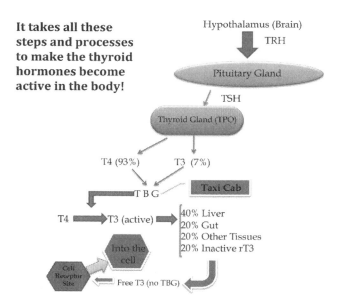

It takes all these steps and processes to make the thyroid hormones become active in the body!

The thyroid is the *master gland* of your metabolism, so it has a crucial job. People who suffer from thyroid malfunction experience many different kinds of health complications, affecting many different systems in their bodies. Every cell in your body has thyroid hormone receptor sites, so this little gland affects the function of every cell in your body!

An estimated twenty-seven million Americans suffer from thyroid dysfunction, half of which goes undiagnosed.[26] Women are at an estimated twenty-four times greater risk of developing thyroid malfunction. The risk of developing thyroid malfunction increases with age for women. Having thyroid dysfunction in your family history also increases your risk for developing thyroid issues. When the thyroid gland begins to malfunction, many doctors neglect to ask the very important question *why*. Adrenal problems, hormonal imbalances, poor blood sugar metabolism, irregular immune function, and gut infections are all signals that the thyroid might be depressed.

Many times replacement hormones are used in an effort to wipe out symptoms, without understanding what has caused the thyroid to malfunction in the first place. More often than not, the relief these drugs provide is short-lived, or never actually works. In order to really address the health of the very important thyroid gland, the systems of the entire body must be taken into account. Just using thyroid replacement hormone in the treatment of low thyroid symptoms ignores most of the steps discussed above.

So even though you are taking medications for thyroid dysfunction, you may still have problems with your thyroid (even though your thyroid stimulating hormone (TSH) levels are in normal range). For example, you can have problems with how the thyroid hormones are transported. Or you can have a problem with how inactive T4 hormone is converted to active T3 hormone. You may have issues with the end effect the thyroid is intended to have at the cell level.

There are six major thyroid patterns that can be tested with thyroid blood tests. When I say thyroid blood tests, I don't just mean testing TSH and T4. In order to really evaluate these six major patterns, a *full thyroid blood panel* needs to be ordered. Later in this chapter, I will list which tests are imperative. To further complicate things, there are twenty-four known patterns of low thyroid function, *many of which need testing other than thyroid blood tests.* Only one thyroid pattern is effectively treated with medication. Once you understand why this concept is true, you will begin to see the folly of considering medication for any other pattern.

Unfortunately, the concept of using thyroid medication and only monitoring two blood indices (TSH and T4) is a 1960's version of treatment. It is extremely outdated. The modern approach is to be aware of the various abnormal body function patterns and the underlying physiological mechanisms that can cause the other five patterns of thyroid trouble.

The first pattern is primary hypothyroidism. In primary hypothyroidism, the thyroid gland gets sort of lazy, and the pituitary gland rushes in by pumping extra TSH in an attempt to prompt the thyroid to produce more thyroid hormones.[27] Primary hypothyroidism affects the entire body. A person may begin to feel sluggish, though there are various symptoms that can occur.

In the second pattern, the TSH will be low, but not as low as with primary hypothyroidism. The pituitary gland, through various mechanisms, fails to produce proper quantities of TSH, so the thyroid gland is not stimulated adequately to produce T4 and T3.[28] Pituitary dysfunction commonly occurs as a result of chronic stress. Chronic stress fatigues the pituitary gland.

The third pattern is thyroid under-conversion. Underconversion occurs when the thyroid gland is making enough T4, but the conversion to T3 is inadequate; therefore, there is low T3. A common reason for inadequate conversion from T4 to T3 can be chronic infection or inflammation.[29] Increased cortisol from the adrenal gland that is responding to stress from a chronic infection may also cause T4 to T3 conversion problems. High cortisol is also toxic to the temporal lobe of the brain, causing poor memory and mental fogginess. The thyroid under-conversion pattern is often missed because low T3 doesn't affect TSH levels, and T3 is rarely checked by the standard blood tests performed by medical physicians. A clue to this pattern is that all other thyroid tests are normal except for T3.[30]

The fourth pattern to cause low thyroid symptoms is thyroid over-conversion of T4 into T3. This seemingly contradictory pattern is possible due to decreased thyroxine-binding globulin (TBG). This pattern occurs when too much T3 is made, and it is overwhelming the cells. The number one cause of this pattern, especially in women, is high blood sugar (glucose) due to resistance to insulin.[31] When someone has insulin resistance their blood glucose will typically be found in the 100–126 milligrams (mg) per deciliter (dl) and higher range [the functional normal is 85-100 milligrams (mg) per deciliter (dl)]. Increased blood glucose causes increased testosterone levels in females, resulting in too much free T3 and too little TBG. Insulin resistance, due to over-consumption of carbohydrates, is also a very common cause of polycystic ovarian syndrome (PCOS) and subsequent difficulty with infertility.[32] Many women who are having difficulty conceiving or maintaining a pregnancy have a thyroid disorder.[33]

The fifth pattern is TBG elevation, which occurs when there is too much TBG in the blood, and too little T3. When TBG is too high, it is like having too many taxicabs for the T3 hormone, and the cabs won't let their passengers out, for fear that they won't get another fare. The TBG elevation pattern is mainly caused by oral contraceptives. Oral contraceptives, or estrogen replacement therapy, cause an increase in estrogen, which then leads to increases in TBG.[34]

The sixth pattern is thyroid resistance. Chronic stress is the root cause of this pattern. Chronic stress stimulates the adrenal glands, which in turn produce far too much cortisol. High levels of cortisol from the adrenal glands cause cells throughout the body to become resistant to thyroid hormones. The pituitary and thyroid are all right, but the hormones are not getting into the cells, thus creating low thyroid symptoms.[35]

Many systems and functions of the body become involved when thyroid function is inadequate, including bone metabolism, the immune system, the nervous system, the endocrine system, gastrointestinal function, liver and gall bladder, growth and sex hormones, fat burning, insulin and glucose metabolism, healthy cholesterol levels, and proper stomach acid.

Sometimes the thyroid gland will not produce enough hormones, which is called hyposecretion. On the other hand, it can produce too many hormones, which is termed hypersecretion. A delicate balance of normal thyroid hormone secretion levels must be kept. If, for example, there is a hyposecretion of the thyroid gland, the nervous system will be affected, and the person will have mental dulling, depression, and memory impairment. If there is a hypersecretion of the thyroid gland, then a person will experience irritability, restlessness, and moodiness. In the cardiovascular system, hyposecretion will cause low heart rate and blood pressure, and hypersecretion will cause rapid heart rate and possible palpitations.[36] The thyroid is so important that when it malfunctions, you will find that many of your systems are influenced.

The bottom line is that poor testing leads to poor results. If the diagnosis is incorrect, then the treatment will be ineffective. More often than not, a TSH test is ordered to evaluate thyroid function, but there are many other tests to consider when understanding the condition of your thyroid. In order to know the underlying cause of your thyroid malfunction, I must run the proper tests. Below is a list of tests that can be a much more accurate reflection of thyroid function:

❖ Total T4: Thyroxin (inactive thyroid hormone)
❖ Total T3: Triiodothyroxine (the active thyroid hormone)
❖ FTI: Free thyroxin index, amount of T4 available
❖ FT4: Free thyroxin (non-protein-bound, inactive thyroid hormones)
❖ T3 uptake: How much of T3 is taken up by TBG
❖ TBG levels: The protein "taxi" that shuttles T4 and T3 around the body

❖ FT3: Free triiodothyroxine (non-protein-bound active thyroid hormones)

❖ Reverse T3: The body cannot use this hormone for metabolism

❖ TPO and TBG Antibodies: Indicator of Hashimoto's Disease

❖ TSI and TR antibodies: Indicators of Graves' Disease

If you have an autoimmune attack on your thyroid gland, then this immune system challenge becomes the *highest priority* of testing and treatment. Handling immune system imbalances requires specialized testing and treatment by a doctor who has been thoroughly trained in the correct protocols. Fortunately for you, I am one of those doctors. I have received in-depth training, and have specialized thyroid dysfunction training from Dr. Datis Kharrazian, who is a respected and highly educated chiropractic physician. Dr. Kharrazian wrote the bestselling book, *Why Do I Still Have Thyroid Symptoms? When My Lab Tests are Normal*. For more information, visit www.thyroidbook.com.

The first thing I have to do is run a complete metabolic profile, which includes a complete thyroid profile. I must also test for vitamin D levels (both active and storage form), anemia, and kidney and liver function. The second factor I need to check is immune imbalance. You must be given an adrenal stress index test along with a food sensitivity test checking for immune reactions to various proteins, such as proteins found in wheat, rye and barley (gluten, various gliadins, wheat germ agglutinin, etc.), casein (milk protein), soy protein, yeast, and eggs. It's imperative that you be tested for gluten sensitivity genes or celiac genes. So far I have not found one patient with thyroid issues that was not genetically susceptible to gluten intolerance. Then I must check for gut infections and the possibility of parasites or yeast. Other factors related to digestive system health must be measured, remembering that 20 percent of T4 to T3 conversion occurs in the gut.

In order to understand the reason why thorough testing is necessary with stubborn thyroid symptoms, you need to remember your thyroid gland influences many body functions. Conversely many systems of the body impact the thyroid gland function. This two-way street is often referred to as thyroid cross talk. Using a whole body approach in regards to testing helps uncover the cause of your thyroid problem. In my opinion it is the only way to fully evaluate this often complex disorder so that your stubborn thyroid symptoms have a successful resolution.

Once the results from your specific lab tests are evaluated and analyzed as a group, I will develop your Johnson Neuro-Metabolic treatment plan around four *key* elements. I will dive into your **diet**, to eliminate those foods that may be contributing to your condition. Certain herbs and foods can have a negative effect on the balance of your immune system. Specific dietary advice will be given to you, so I can improve your immune system balance.

Then I must detail any **lifestyle changes** that are necessary to reduce stress on various body systems and glands.

Along with diet and lifestyle changes, there are **specific nutritional supplements** that must be taken in order to facilitate healing and recovery. The consumption of these nutritional supplements will ensure that the repair process goes smoothly, and that the immune system is brought back into balance.

Finally, if indicated, I will use a customized and carefully monitored **Johnson Brain-Based Therapy** protocol designed especially for you, based on your functional neurological examination. Johnson Brain-Based Therapy is how I help your body bring itself back into balance so it can heal the causes of your thyroid symptoms. By using my comprehensive approach, I get to the bottom of your pain, ill health, brain fog, and bodily imbalance.

Below I have listed some very important influences of thyroid hormones on physiological and metabolic function.

❖ **Bone**: Deficiency of thyroid hormones leads to a decrease in bone development and an abnormal architecture of the bone is created. Generally, a functionally low (which means low but not flagged as of yet) serum calcium is noted in hypothyroidism. Elevated thyroid hormones cause increased serum calcium, as they pull calcium from the bone, leading to increased risk of pathological fractures of the spine and weight bearing joints.

❖ **Gastrointestinal Function**: Transit time is affected directly by thyroid hormones, as is the absorption of nutrients.

❖ **Male Hormones**: Hypothyroidism has been linked to diminished libido and impotence. Although hypothyroidism is more rare in men, it must be considered in treating these conditions.

❖ **Liver and Gall Bladder Function**: Low thyroid function causes decreased liver clearance of hormones and other metabolites as well as gall bladder congestion through thickening of the bile, often also associated with an elevation of cholesterol. Unfortunately, cholesterol elevation (the symptom) is often treated with cholesterol lowering drugs, while the thyroid function as the cause of the elevated cholesterol is ignored.

❖ **Body Composition**: As you may know all too well, low thyroid function causes an inability to lose weight, which is caused by a slowed conversion of glucose and fat into energy, and an alteration of the way human growth hormone (HGH) is metabolized in the body.

❖ **Blood Sugar Regulation**: Low thyroid slows the insulin response to glucose following the eating of carbohydrates or sugar, and it also slows glucose uptake into cells and tissues, and slows absorption of glucose from the intestinal tract. In other words, your entire energy production system is slowed. It is quite confounding to your body and brain, in that the glucose is in the blood, but the tissues are not able to absorb it. Thyroid related blood sugar regulation really confuses the pituitary gland and adrenal glands, resulting in a "stress physiology," even if life is good.

❖ **Cholesterol**: As mentioned earlier, low thyroid increases your cholesterol and triglycerides, so your doctor tells you your diet is poor. You become even more strict in your diet, and the tissue starvation (low glucose, low energy) gets worse, which makes the stress physiology worse, which makes your cholesterol higher, which prompts your doctor to put you on cholesterol medication. All cholesterol medications interfere with energy production because they block the formation of coenzyme Q10 (CoQ10). Coenzyme Q10 is produced by all cells and is needed for the cell to make adenosine triphosphate (ATP) molecules. ATP is considered by biologists to be the energy currency of life. This cascade of events further stresses your body function, and can lead to major frustration with your health.

❖ **Depression**: Low thyroid impairs the production of stimulating neurotransmitters, which are the chemicals that antidepressants work on. Low stimulating neurotransmitters leave you feeling, as one of my professors described, "lower than a snake's belly."

❖ **Female Hormones**: Low thyroid changes the way estrogen is metabolized in the body, shifting toward an estrogen metabolite that has been proven to increase the risk of breast cancer.

❖ **Stress**: Low thyroid slows the elimination of the stress hormone, cortisol, which leaves you feeling stressed-out, not because of stress, but because the stress hormone can't be removed efficiently.

❖ **Detoxification**: Low thyroid slows an enzyme critical for metabolic biotransformation, or detoxification, the process by which the body binds and removes all environmental chemicals and normal byproducts of metabolism, including hormones. "Toxicity" further slows your metabolism, and leads to headaches and other toxic symptoms.

❖ **Digestion**: Low thyroid reduces the release of Gastrin, which determines the output of hydrochloric acid in the stomach, leading to poor protein digestion, sour stomach, and gastroesophageal reflux disease (GERD).

❖ **Thermoregulation**: Regulation of body temperature is affected by low thyroid, resulting in hot flashes and night sweats, which is especially prominent in pre-menopausal women. Temperature regulation difficulty is often blamed on estrogen dropping, but may be directly caused by low thyroid.

❖ **PMS and Infertility**: Low thyroid affects the progesterone receptors, making them less sensitive to progesterone, which feels like low progesterone although progesterone levels may be normal. Since the activity of progesterone is diminished, the health of the uterus is insufficient for implantation in the second half of the female cycle, leading to difficulties getting pregnant, and to premenstrual syndrome (PMS). Low thyroid also reduces sex hormone binding proteins, leading to an increase in estrogen activity.

❖ **<u>Anemia</u>**: Low thyroid affects protein metabolism, which then lowers the red blood cell mass that carries oxygen to tissues for metabolism of energy. Yes, another mechanism for feeling lousy.

❖ **<u>Homocysteine</u>**: Low thyroid slows a process called methylation, often evidenced by elevated serum levels of homocysteine. Elevated homocysteine in the blood has been proven as a risk factor for cardiovascular disease, Alzheimer's and other neurodegenerative disorders, and cervical dysplasia.

As you can see, living with low thyroid has *far-reaching* repercussions on your health and function. There are as many as twenty-four published mechanisms for thyroid function to be impaired. When you have symptoms of low thyroid, but you have been told you are fine, take charge and get a more complete set of tests. You need to get the *right diagnosis* to truly heal the cause of your thyroid symptoms in order to protect your health.

TESTIMONIALS

"I feel clearer, my thought processes are better, I have more energy, and it's as if the body has finally said, 'oh I'm so pleased with myself now!'"

"I've lived in different parts of the world throughout my life, and have had health issues on and off. The thing that was most concerning to me was my thyroid, because I was diagnosed with hypothyroidism. I tried to stay on the natural health side of things instead of getting into allopathic medicine. I was quite successful up to a point, but not feeling 100 percent. I had come to Dr. Johnson before, and he was most helpful with other issues. Then I tried Armour, and that caused some interesting issues with my eye. I was diagnosed with no problems as far as my eyes were concerned, but instead diagnosed with hypothyroidism (with elevated levels of TSH).

So I decided to come back to Dr. Johnson, because he seemed the most wise and sensible, to me, in his approach. He ran blood tests that showed my immune system antibodies to my thyroid were extremely high. In fact, he said he's never seen a number like that. He had other tests prescribed for me, and I discovered that I have milk and gluten intolerance. The tests also showed that I was within the parameters of having celiac.

Having gone through what he already prescribed for me, dealing with my thyroid, I have felt so much better. My body doesn't feel bloated all the time. I feel clearer, my thought processes are better, I have more energy, and it's as if the body has finally said, 'Oh, I'm so pleased with myself now! I'm on the right track, so let's continue!' Every time I come, things just look more positive, and I feel I'm on the right road. Dr. Johnson and his staff have just been marvelous!"

-Astrid Ganson, Dearborn, MI

"Helping A Patient with Graves' Disease Naturally..."

"I've been a patient of Dr. Johnson's for a very long time, at least seventeen years. Earlier this year, in mid-February, I was diagnosed with Graves' disease, an autoimmune disease that relates thyroid issues with eye issues. I had hyperthyroidism, so my thyroid gland was producing too much of TSH thyroid hormone. I explored it through eye doctors and went to an endocrinologist, and he put me on thyroid medication, which was a thyroid blocker, to stop my thyroid from producing too much. It was that, or I would have to get rid of my thyroid and be on medication for the rest of my life, and I wasn't ready for that option.

I started the medication, and in the meantime I was exploring this autoimmune issue with Dr. Johnson. When he saw my blood work, he said that I had an autoimmune issue, but he suspected maybe celiac, because if I had that gene it would be near the thyroid gene, and that could be why the autoimmune issue was attacking my thyroid.

I was on the thyroid medication while Dr. Johnson and I were exploring this, and I did the tests that he recommended, to see if my body built antibodies to gluten, soy, dairy, and yeast. Well, I had an issue with every single one of them! As soon as I found that out, I decided to just take that all out of my diet, and I have learned a lot since then too. Some of the things that I thought were gluten free have hidden things in them, but Dr. Johnson has given me a ton of information such as websites, lists of foods to eat, dietary ideas, and recipes, so I could learn more about what else to stay away from. Within three months of just not eating those foods, I was off of my thyroid medication, which made me extremely happy, since I don't like being on medication.

I decided to do one of his programs, the six-month one. It is very comprehensive and includes diet, supplements, and all kinds of treatment programs. Since I started the program, which has been just over a month, I have noticed many changes. I had a rash on my ankle from the Graves' disease, which is totally gone. I had knee pain in my left knee when I would remain idle, and that is also completely gone. I used to stand up from my desk and limp for the first minute, until my knee warmed up. I had symptoms of a racing heart probably one to two times a day, three to four times a week, and within the last month, I have only noticed this happen twice. I've noticed a difference, and had less stomach bloating and gas. I've noticed all of these things within the month, along with being off my meds. I'm thrilled, and can't wait to continue all of the things I have been doing."

-Mary Cieslak, Rochester, MI

"Her Doctor Said Her Lab Tests Were 'Normal'... But Thanks To Dr. Johnson..."

"I had been feeling down all the time, and had no energy—I really felt like 'doggie doo doo!' I slept nine to ten hours per night and still felt tired, and I gained weight. My medical doctor said I was okay. He increased my thyroid medication, and I went downhill from there. Then I saw a specialist, who ran a lot of blood tests and told me I was fine.

I told my chiropractor in Richmond, and he sent me to Dr. Johnson, who he said could help me. Dr. Johnson examined me using Contact Reflex Analysis (CRA), and prescribed several nutritional supplements. Now, almost four months later, I feel fine. I have my energy back, and can do things I couldn't do before, like karate and staying up after 10:00 p.m. I'm also sleeping only six hours a day, and feel rested and energized. My body once again feels like it's functioning properly. Thanks, Dr. Johnson!"

-S. G., Richmond, MI

"I'm More Upbeat And My Hair Isn't Falling Out, Thanks To Dr. Johnson"

"About a year ago, my medical doctor told me that my thyroid (TSH and T4) was low. Since I've been a practice member since 1994, I immediately told Dr. Johnson about the problem.

Dr. Johnson recommended supplements directly related to thyroid. I've taken them regularly, and recently had my annual physical. I'm happy to report that everything was normal. I have more energy since taking the supplements. Also, I'm more upbeat and my hair isn't falling out any more.

I still take the thyroid supplements; however, the amount has been greatly reduced over the last few months. Thanks, Dr. J, for helping my thyroid problem without drugs."

-Ramona Meirow, Romeo, MI

CHAPTER 9

Peripheral Neuropathy

Peripheral neuropathy (PN) describes damage to the peripheral nervous system (PNS), the vast communications network that transmits information from the brain and spinal cord (the central nervous system) to every other part of the body. Peripheral nerves also send sensory information back to the brain and spinal cord, such as a message that the feet are cold or that a finger is burned. Damage to the peripheral nervous system interferes with these vital connections.

Patients with peripheral neuropathy often experience chronic tingling, numbness, weakness, or burning pain, most often in the legs and/or feet, but these symptoms can also occur in the arms or hands. Due to poor sensation coming from the legs and feet, those with PN often find many things difficult. They find it difficult to walk, to sense if they are going down stairs properly, or know if they have injured the affected area, and generally they are miserable because of the chronic pain they often experience.

Neuropathy can be caused by many things, such as an under-firing of the part of the brain called the parietal lobe, side effects from certain medications, or complications from sugar imbalances. The result is burning, numbness, or tingling.

In the brain, there is a road map of your entire body. Your feet, your hands, and your face are all represented in the parietal lobe. If poor nerve signals come into the brain because of peripheral neuropathy, problems arise in the brain. The brain and nerves need constant stimulation for them to stay alive and do their job, which is to send and receive messages.

Although you might start out with peripheral neuropathy, the longer you have this condition, the more likely you will experience issues higher up in other areas of the brain. Malfunction higher up in the brain is why damage to the peripheral nerves is just a part of the story, and why treating the local area can lead to short-term and discouraging results.

What is so dangerous about peripheral neuropathy is that it is not an injury like a broken bone or a scrape. Numbness usually comes on slowly. You don't notice it at first, or maybe you just brush off the sensation, thinking that it is nothing. Slowly it begins to build, and you start feeling numbness and tingling. You become more irritable. You start taking pills to get through the day, to function at work, or to run your errands. One day you realize that you are not the same person you used to be, and then you make an appointment with your family doctor. When it comes to a condition like peripheral neuropathy, many doctors just don't have the training or experience to properly diagnose the true cause of your problem.

Peripheral neuropathy is a tricky condition. Your numbness and tingling can have a number of causes, and some of these causes are not even in the area where you are experiencing the numbness or tingling. Because many doctors don't know where these places are, they assume that since your numbness or tingling is in your wrist, hand, arm, leg, or foot, the problem is solely in that region. Going to your family doctor may cause your condition to become more severe. Worse yet, you may receive surgery for it.

The biggest problem with the treatments that some doctors prescribe for peripheral neuropathy is that they go after your symptoms and treat them with medications. Some doctors give their patients anti-seizure medications like Neurotin for their neuropathy. Anti-seizure medications like Neurotin, Klonopin, and Topamax were not meant to cure neuropathy. These drugs were developed for epilepsy, and they work by using a chemical that tells your brain to slow down. Using medications may be alright once in a while, however anti-seizure medications for PN can only make your condition worse in the long run, in two very specific ways.

First, the numbness, burning, and tingling are your body's way of telling you that there is something wrong. Because you feel numbness, burning, or tingling, you stop doing the things that can make your problem worse. But if you are taking pills so you can get through a day of work, you are probably making your problem worse because you've sabotaged your body's only means of keeping you healthy. Medication is *not* a permanent fix. No matter how many pills you take, you will never truly heal.

Secondly, these pills can cause dangerous side effects. The chemicals they disable do more than just slow down your brain. Depending on what pill you are taking, you can leave yourself open to liver failure, kidney damage, and gastrointestinal hemorrhage. These side effects are one hundred times worse than the numbness and tingling that you are taking these pills for in the first place.

Wrist or foot splints are another common treatment sometimes prescribed for muscle weakness accompanying peripheral neuropathy. Frequently, the user may wear the splints for more hours than necessary, thinking more is better. Wearing wrist or foot splints may seem harmless enough, but you're only supposed to wear them for the specified time. Using splints as a crutch will lead to scar tissue formation in your wrist or foot, which can complicate treatment.

Since none of your doctor's treatments are meant to actually correct the true cause of your problem, these treatments are most likely making you worse. You will be wearing your splint longer and longer, and your pills will have to get stronger and stronger. The quality of your life will undoubtedly begin to lower.

After you have been given the pills and the splints, you will most likely receive physical therapy. The problem with physical therapy is that the therapists only follow the directions given by your doctor. If your doctor has not discovered the true cause of your condition, then the physical therapist continues to work on the part of the body where you feel numbness, burning, and tingling. Since the root cause of your PN is not being addressed, your treatment leaves you feeling disappointed and hopeless.

If none of these treatments work, doctors usually tell their patients to learn to live with it. I am here to tell you that a life doomed to PN doesn't have to be your reality. If your doctor's treatments fail, it doesn't mean that you are incurable. It means that your doctor was likely looking in the wrong place. The majority of doctors tend to get so sidetracked by focusing on the area involved that they overlook something so incredibly obvious.

You see, in order for any sensation to travel to your brain, it has to find a pathway. In essence, it needs a road to get there, just like you need a road to get to your job in the morning. In your body, this road is called the nervous system. If you interfere with the nervous system anywhere along its path, it can make you feel numbness, burning, or tingling in places like your wrist, hands, arms, legs, and feet.

So if all this attention your doctor has given to the area of numbness, burning, and tingling doesn't seem to make any difference in your recovery, it may be because there is nothing wrong with that body part at all.

If you are suffering from constant, bothersome paresthesia (altered sensation), or maybe you feel a slight numbness, burning, or tingling that you do not want to get worse, then there is hope for you. I take a comprehensive approach to helping my patients with peripheral neuropathy. Not only do I treat the local area affected by using cutting edge therapy and addressing metabolic conditions, but I also treat the areas in the brain responsible for receiving these messages from the body.

It is possible that peripheral nerve damage will lead to functional changes in the brain, so all areas must be addressed in order to get the best outcomes. I get results by looking at you with a fresh set of diagnostic and therapeutic eyes. At my treatment center, I have combined five key elements, what I like to call ingredients, to address and properly heal the damaged nerves in your feet and hands. Used together, these five key elements provide true and lasting relief from neuropathy. Just as in a recipe, if you leave out an ingredient, or don't put in the right amounts of the ingredients, you don't get the results you are looking for.

These five key elements are:

- Functional peripheral nerve evaluation

- Peripheral nerve stimulation
- Biomedical nerve nutrition
- Increase cellular energy and adenosine triphosphate (ATP) [the energy currency the body makes to sustain life] in the nerve
- Peripheral balance feedback coordination

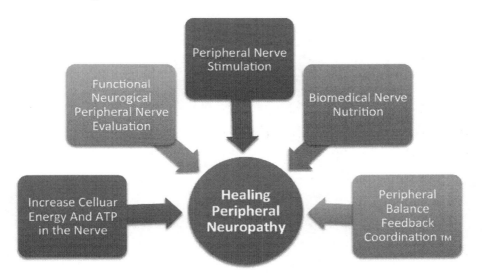

Most neuropathy treatment approaches include one or maybe two of these key elements in healing peripheral neuropathy, while completely ignoring the others. I use a combination of these key elements based on your specific condition, and address peripheral neuropathy in a very dynamic way.

As with all the chronic conditions mentioned in this book, I want to help you heal from the inside out. I can help to heal you with our Johnson Neuro-Metabolic Treatment plan, so that you have long-term success in your healing process. The approaches I use are effective and thorough. The one size fits all mentality has no place in my work. When you come to me with numbness, tingling, or pain, I will get to the very bottom of what is not functioning in your body, and then I will create a plan specifically for you. Working together with you, I can help you turn around your peripheral neuropathy and alleviate your chronic pain.

Conclusion

I often close my public educational seminars and webinars by asking if the participants believe the following statement is true:

Knowledge is Power

Most of the audience members confidently nod their heads up and down, agreeing that it is a true statement. I pause for a few moments, and boldly state that I don't believe it is true. A few more moments pass, and I assert the following corollary of this concept to be true:

Knowledge is Only Potential Power…It's Not Worth *Anything* Unless You Use it!

I'm sure you know where I am headed with this line of thought. It's important that I do "go there." Suffering with a chronic condition is not fun. It's frustrating, to say the least, and more likely, disheartening. Watching others do the things you only wish you could do again, and trying to remember the past when you felt like a fully functioning human being, is demoralizing. So yes, I must prod you to take action.

You have probably lost hope like most of the patients I have seen over the years with chronic health challenges. It takes a lot of coaxing to help patients, like you, take the necessary action steps toward the healing journey that can change your circumstances. With that in mind, ask yourself the following questions honestly, and consider writing down your answers:

1. How much has your health challenge affected your job, relationships, finances, family, and other activities?
2. What has your health challenge cost you in terms of time, money, happiness, and freedom?
3. Where do you picture yourself in one to three years if your health challenge isn't handled?
4. What is it worth for you to be able to live your life without your health challenge being such a burden?

Take some time to digest your responses. Think about the *quality of your life*, and what you want for yourself. You may think that you just have to learn to live with your condition. You may have been told that you will never recover, and that your condition will only get worse. But what if it were possible to be 30 percent, 50 percent, 80 percent better? What about 100 percent? What would your life be like then? What would be a deal breaker, in other words, is there anything you would not do, to be able to regain an improved quality of life?

I want you to know that there is *hope*, and that you most likely can improve your health. I specialize in helping frustrated people who have chronic conditions reorganize and heal their lives. Johnson Neuro-Metabolic Therapy may be the answer to your chronic condition. Our blend of *state of the art treatments and diagnostic methods gets* to the underlying cause of your condition. When the cause of your health challenge is identified and removed, your body can begin the miraculous healing process, so that you can get back to the life you dream of living!

Even people who have been to the Mayo Clinic, searching for answers and coming up empty-handed, have benefited from our new and exciting treatments.

My guess is that you have not had a doctor who is as thorough in their evaluation, nor have you had a doctor who actually understands you the way that I do. You need a doctor who actually looks at all the underlying mechanisms creating dysfunction, a doctor who is *not* going to shove prescription medications down your throat that rob you of your personality, making you feel like a zombie, numb to the world. There is a healthier, more thorough and effective way, I assure you.

Please understand, however, that I can't help everyone, which is why I thoroughly evaluate every patient who comes into our office. I have to determine whether you are a candidate for this very special care. The method by which I determine if you are a candidate for our care is to obtain a case review. When you think about it you have two options when it comes to your improving your health:

1. Do the same things you have been doing: eat the same things, see the same doctors, take the same medications... and hope for different results.

2. Do something different. Different may be new. Different may be scary. But different produces what kind of result? NEW AND DIFFERENT.

Johnson Neuro-Metabolic Therapy could be the start to your new life! Now is the time for you to take control of your health. I invite you to contact me for a thorough evaluation, so I may discuss all the possibilities of regaining your health and **reclaiming your life**!

Critical Reading For What's Next

Chronic health challenge triggers are as individual as snowflakes, and the first task at hand is gaining a thorough understanding of the underlying issue(s). As explained throughout this book, once I get a handle on the factors leading to your deteriorated health, I can develop an individualized treatment program.

Below I have listed the specific tests and therapies I currently offer at our center to put you on the path of true healing. You will recognize some of the descriptions from the fibromyalgia chapter. I've expanded the list here so you can have a ready reference in one location. I determine which of these tests and treatments to use on a case-by-case basis.

❖ **Comprehensive thyroid panels (10 specific lab tests)**
❖ **A complete metabolic panel (CMP):** The CMP allows us to check your blood glucose levels, since glucose and oxygen are needed by the brain to function properly.

As part of the CMP, I obtain tests for inflammation in your system by testing homocysteine levels, C-Reactive Protein (C-RP), and other markers such as erythrocyte sedimentation rate (ESR), low triglycerides, fibrinogen, etc.

Just about every chronic condition patient I have treated suffers from some form of chronic inflammatory process.

❖ **A complete lipid panel:** This test shows your cholesterol and triglyceride levels, as well as HDL ("good cholesterol") and LDL ("bad cholesterol"). When levels of these lipids are too high *or* too low I am alerted to various body function imbalances that need to be addressed.

❖ **A CBC (complete blood chemistry with auto differential):** Red blood cells help me understand your oxygen carrying capacity. In addition, the immune system function is represented in the white blood cells with this panel of markers.

❖ **Adrenal Stress Index (ASI):** I test adrenal gland function with a test called Adrenal Stress Index. The primary chemical I am testing with the ASI is cortisol. The ASI is a salivary test, much like DNA testing.

Your adrenal glands are your "stress" organs, meaning that they react to stress. If you have been or are currently under stress (and who isn't if you have a chronic health challenge?), this test is a must. If you have Stage 7 adrenal gland exhaustion, you will experience blood sugar spikes and valleys that make nerve cells unstable, and could be the reason you have fibromyalgia, migraines, or other chronic conditions.

Often, elevated nighttime cortisol levels will lead to insomnia. When your body's cortisol levels are abnormal, you will suffer from insomnia and hormonal imbalances. Cortisol levels can be corrected via specific nutritional and lifestyle-change protocols, thereby bringing balance back to itself, and making you feel alive and alert again.

❖ **Immune Panels**: Your condition could be caused by an autoimmune disorder. As you know, an autoimmune disorder is where your immune system attacks a particular area of the body (nervous system, joints, connective tissue, thyroid, etc.).

Specific imbalances that occur when the immune system is in the "attack mode" can be measured. The information provided by this test guides my recommendations for nutritional supplementation and dietary changes to help bring balance back to the immune system. A specialized lab enables us to test for specific antibodies to determine if you suffer from an autoimmune condition, and specify what tissues are in the cross hairs of your immune system. Very valuable knowledge indeed!

❖ **Neurotransmitters**: I test for decreased chemical messengers called brain neurotransmitters. Neurotransmitters are vital for proper brain function.

Decreased neurotransmitters can cause increased pain. Neurotransmitter imbalance can lead to the many emotional symptoms the chronic pain patient experiences. Neurotransmitters don't cross the blood-brain barrier; that is to say, they stay in a separated blood partition in the brain. As a result, I use questionnaires to help us understand your neurotransmitter balance.

❖ **Hormone Panels**: I can check hormone panels to determine if you suffer from low testosterone (in males) or low estrogen/progesterone levels (in females). Conversely, males can have estrogen levels that are too high, and women can have testosterone levels that are too high. Symptoms related to hormone levels that are altered from what is normal may include depression, fatigue, mental fogginess, mood swings, hot flashes, sweating attacks, weight gain, decreased physical stamina, and many thyroid symptoms, due to the cross talk between the thyroid and the endocrine (hormone) system.

❖ **Sensitivity Testing**: Many patients with chronic conditions have food sensitivities, or worse, an immune reaction to gluten (a peptide found in wheat, rye and barley, and their derivatives) caused by an inherited gene. I can also test you for foods that "look like" gluten to the immune system, which can also cause the same or similar reactions as gluten. Having these sensitivities causes the gut to be inflamed, which in turn causes brain inflammation. It is important to note that gut inflammation is characterized by bloating, not pain. The predominant symptom for brain inflammation is brain fog: just what many fibromyalgia and chronic pain and chronic condition sufferers experience regularly.

❖ **Gastrointestinal Functional Analysis**: Proper gastrointestinal (GI) function is critical to adequate nutritional status, and can impact all aspects of body function. The profiles tested address key components of proper GI health, including measurement of beneficial microbial flora, opportunistic bacteria, yeast, and parasitic infection. The presence of abnormal disease causing bacteria (including H. Pylori), or imbalance of the over four hundred normal bacterial strains in the gut, can cause gut inflammation. Having yeast overgrowth, parasites, fungi, or other undesirable vermin in your digestive tract can cause many of the health challenges thyroid, fibromyalgia, and other chronic health sufferers experience, such as joint pain or brain fog. These unwanted invaders can also lead to an autoimmune attack in your body. This DNA test is supersensitive, and often is a very important piece of the diagnostic puzzle that will finally help with the resolution of your health challenge. In addition, markers of inflammation, immune function, and digestion and absorption are measured with this comprehensive test.

❖ **Increased Intestinal Permeability or "Leaky Gut" Testing**: Your intestines are supposed to allow the entry of good healthy food particles and nutrients into your body, and act as a shield to substances that are not wanted or needed, or which are damaging to the body. When your digestive tract has been damaged from inflammation or other causes, it can leak like a sieve. Conversely, your digestive tract can be so badly damaged that hardly any nourishment can come into the body, as in advanced celiac disease. The blood test we order is the newest method of determining autoimmune attack of specific intestinal cell components, and it allows me to know whether you have leaky gut syndrome (LGS), which is also known as intestinal barrier dysfunction. In addition to the above-mentioned problems LGS causes, LGS will also cause damage to your health, due to allergy reactions and immune reactions to the unwanted particles that make it into your bloodstream. Even your brain and nervous system health will be affected with leaky gut syndrome. One recent study shows the inflammation from LGS plays a role in the development of major depression.[37] LGS adds insult to injury, and needs to be addressed if you are to recover your health. The only way to see if you have LGS is to test for it. I am thorough, so I perform this test, for your health's sake.

Johnson Brain–Based Therapy Improves Imbalances Found in Your Nervous System

The foundation of all of our treatment programs, no matter what the chronic health condition, lies in this truth: *Every cell in your body, especially your brain and nervous system, needs two things to survive.* Those two things are:

❖ Fuel – in the form of oxygen and glucose

❖ Activation – nerve cells need proper stimulation, or else they degenerate and die

It is very important for you to know how important fuel is, especially balanced blood sugar and oxygen, when you suffer from a chronic illness.

❖ **Balanced Blood Sugar**: Glucose comes from the foods you eat. Your brain must have enough glucose, but does not like blood sugar swings. Overeating of sugar and high carbohydrate foods is epidemic. Abusing carbohydrates leads to massive blood sugar swings, with hypoglycemia (excessively low) as one extreme, and diabetes as the other. Your brain cannot work properly that way...but I can help you with your sugar balance.

❖ **Oxygen**: After about age twenty, *you lose your ability to use oxygen* by 1 percent per year. So, for example, at age forty-seven, you've lost 27 percent of your capacity. Because people's ability to use oxygen goes down with age, I check oxygen levels on all of our patients.

Oxygen is like gasoline in the gas tank of your car. As you get older, having enough oxygen becomes crucial. If you don't have any gas in the car, you are not going anywhere. Oxygen stimulates your nervous system to enhance healing and repair, thus decreasing pain, promoting more restful sleep, and bringing many other health benefits. One focus of our recovery program is to increase your oxygen, so your brain and nervous system can do its job. Without oxygen available for your brain and nervous system, it is quite likely that no treatment will work.

For more information I recommend that you read the book, Energize Your Brain, Change Your Life: An Introduction To Exercise With Oxygen Therapy, by Dr. Jeff Donatello. I am a contributor to this book.

As powerful as oxygen is for healing your body, it's not enough to do the job. Fuel is not enough by itself. Your brain must be stimulated to stay healthy, work correctly,

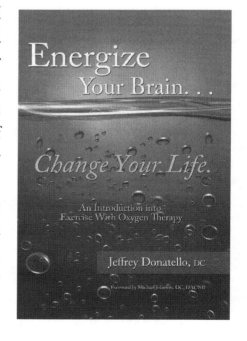

and create healing and balance. Here are just a few of the powerful brain activations I use in our highly successful chronic condition recovery programs to give sufferers just like you the relief you desperately want:

- ❖ **Brain-Based Therapy (BBT)**: A revolutionary breakthrough treatment program pioneered by the country's leading chiropractic neurologist, Dr. Fredrick Carrick. The treatments are all neurologically based, and clinically proven to help with chronic pain, balance disorders, and other neurologic conditions. Brain-based therapy stimulates your body's built in sensors (such as sight, sound, touch and smell), which are wired and connected to the various areas of your brain. So if I find weakened areas in your right parietal lobe, then I am going to use receptors that are wired to the parietal lobe. It is complex. Everything I do is non-invasive, does not use drugs, and promotes proper function in the brain. The brain has an amazing ability to adapt, change, and rewire if I give it the proper fuel and activation. The ability for the brain to rewire itself is termed neuroplasticity. Johnson Brain-Based Therapy is designed to promote positive neuroplasticity in your brain.

Perhaps Dr. Robert Melillo, D.C., states the concept best in his book, *Disconnected Kids:*

Conventional medical wisdom long held that the human brain cannot change—that it is hardwired at birth just like a computer. Scientists started to collect evidence in the early 1970's that eventually proved this is not the case. They found that the brain is actually malleable and has the ability to change both physically and chemically in response to certain types of activity. They found that it can change its shape, size, number of branches, number of connections, as well as the strength of its connections. The potential of this ability is so far reaching, it has become a science of its own called neuroplasticity—*neuro* meaning neurons and *plastic* meaning changeable.[38]

❖ **Auditory Stimulation**: Listening to sound in one ear, with a specially designed earphone (that combines both the right and left channel into a single earbud), will mainly stimulate the opposite side of the brain and increase neurological activity. Different sounds (frequencies, tone, pitches) affect the right and left sides of the brain differently. I use professionally composed music that specifically activates one side of the brain. I use right brain music if your right brain needs stimulation, or left brain music if your left brain needs stimulation.

❖ **Olfactory Stimulation**: Your sense of smell is special. Your sight, sound, taste, and touch all travel through a sensory "middleman" area of your brain called the thalamus. *But smell goes directly to the brain.* There is no middleman. Smells are powerful brain stimulations. I'm sure you've experienced this phenomenon: the smell of homemade cookies baking in the oven suddenly flooding your mind with fond memories of your childhood, and making your mouth water. Or on the other hand, just a whiff of spoiled milk causing your stomach to turn. Smells that appeal to you stimulate the left side of the brain, and smells that offend you stimulate the right side of the brain.

❖ **<u>Calorics</u>**: A small amount of warm water in the ear will stimulate the semicircular canals in your inner ear. Nerves inside the semicircular canals send massive signals through the vestibular nerve, in a chain reaction, to several important brain areas: the cerebellum, the cortex, and then down to the lower brainstem (pontomedullary region). Remember, it is your lower brainstem and cortex that slow down the over-firing upper brainstem (mesencephalon). Caloric stimulation is also fantastic for treating underlying causes of dizziness.

These brain-based therapy treatments are just a few of the methods that I may use to help your brain increase its firing. I have literally over one hundred ways to specifically activate and stimulate the brain. The key to the success of Johnson Brain-Based Rehabilitation is to be extremely specific in diagnosing the weak brain areas and applying activations or stimulations to those specific weakened areas. Other treatments I use involve eye movements, gross motor activities, light therapy, cognitive activities, puzzles, etc. The list is huge, and specific to each individual's needs. Here are a few more:

❖ **Eyelights Therapy**: Eyelights were designed to provide optimal stimulation to the brain using the optic nerve. Glasses designed with flashing lights built to fit behind the lens, can be programmed to blink on the non-dominant eye in order to strengthen the weaker side of the brain. Since one of the most direct avenues to the brain is via the eye, children can learn more effectively if they are seeing correctly. And an athlete will perform better because the eye is able to gather all of the information necessary to perform. By stimulating the weaker hemisphere of the brain, you allow it to become stronger, thus improving overall performance. One method of stimulating the brain is to use light pulses. When using Eyelights you can control the intensity, frequency, and pattern of light pulses, which will result in being able to "wake up" the weaker side of the brain.

❖ **Unilateral Adjusting**: Understanding how and why to specifically adjust areas of the spine or extremities is very important to creating the best possible outcomes. I have been trained in neurologically based adjustments. The right brain controls the left side of the body, and the left brain controls the right side. If there is a decrease of firing or impulses in one side of the brain, I only want to stimulate the joints on the opposite side. Makes sense, doesn't it? Don't worry; I will only use very light instrument activation, so you will not get worse.

Have you ever had a massage, a chiropractic manipulation, or physical therapy, and felt worse afterward? It is because the treatment was too much for your nervous system. It over-stimulated you, and you crashed. As I describe it, it exceeded metabolic capacity (EMC).

❖ **<u>Triton DTS – Non-Surgical Spinal Decompression</u>**: This treatment uses a computer guided system that gently lengthens and decompresses the spine to provide lasting relief from chronic neck and back pain due to disc problems. I was one of the first chiropractic offices to bring non-surgical spinal decompression (NSSD) to Shelby Township. Years of experience have given me a clinical edge, allowing you to get the fastest relief possible.

❖ **<u>ReBuilder</u>**: Not only useful for peripheral neuropathy, this electrical stimulator sends a comfortable electronic pulse/signal to your feet and legs, which can get your nerves functioning again. The ReBuilder™ is theorized to restore, stabilize, and help stimulate rebuilding the nerves in your extremities.

❖ **<u>Interactive Metronome</u>**: This computerized brain-based rehabilitation assessment and training program helps to literally retrain your brain's circuitry. Using the Interactive Metronome helps patients with ADD/ADHD, learning disorders, MS, Parkinson's disease, and stroke rehab (and other health challenges).

The Interactive Metronome is used to reprogram and balance the brain. I am a Certified Interactive Metronome Physician. Visit www.interactivemetronome.com for more information.

❖ **<u>ATM2 System</u>**: One of my favorite tools is this unique exercise device, which provides relief from chronic neck, back, shoulder, and hip pain by restoring core muscle strength. It increases range of motion by reprogramming the central nervous system (CNS) for the proper firing pattern of your muscles. The ATM2 can bring back pain relief in as little as five minutes. Visit www.backproject.com for more information.

❖ **<u>Whole Body Advanced Vibration Exercise (WAVE)</u>**: WAVE is a helpful treatment modality that provides near 100 percent muscle recruitment and strong neurological and circulatory stimulation. In short fifteen-minute sessions, it helps relieve chronic neck and back pain, peripheral and diabetic neuropathy, shoulder, arm, wrist, hip, leg, and foot pain, and adds strength to muscles throughout the body. Using WAVE also helps reverse osteoporosis throughout the body.

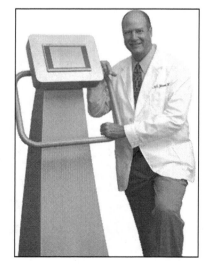

❖ **Cold Laser Therapy (Low Level Laser Therapy or LLLT)**: Using laser in healing is a relatively new occurrence. LLLT therapy is an FDA-cleared treatment that has been shown to decrease pain and inflammation, speed healing, and more. By directing specific frequencies of laser and near infrared light to the body, this painless treatment can accelerate the healing process and increase circulation. LLLT has been clinically shown to help with carpal tunnel syndrome, peripheral neu-

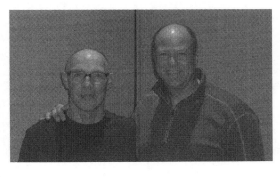

ropathy, RSDS, fibromyalgia, and other painful conditions. I received specialized training for the cold laser from Dr. Jeff Spencer, who was the team doctor for eight consecutive Team U.S.A. Tour De France wins.

In addition to Johnson Neuro-Metabolic Therapy, I also employ services and procedures to "crack the code" on the several aspects of the underlying causes of chronic pain and chronic health challenges, such as:

❖ **Nutritional Counseling**: Part of the bigger picture to restoring your health is how you eat. I have specialized training in the science behind the Blood Type

Diet, among other methods, to provide you with sound direction when it comes to eating well and correctly using nutritional supplementation.

❖ **<u>Glutathione Therapy</u>**: Known as the mother of all antioxidants, glutathione is found in almost every cell in the body. Glutathione can help decrease pain and inflammation, give you more energy, and rid your body of numerous toxins. Glutathione is not well absorbed when taken in pill form, so my protocols use other forms of supplementation.

❖ **<u>Individualized Home Exercise Planning</u>**: The patients that get the best results are those who take an active role in their recovery. I empower you with individualized exercise programs tailored to your specific needs. These plans often contain several "phases" that change as you become stronger and healthier. Let's make you the best you can be! Of special note, I am a Certified Back Power Plus trained physician.

❖ **<u>Computerized Blind Spot Mapping</u>**: I use a computer-based test that measures how well each side of the brain is functioning based on measurement of the size of the patient's blind spot. This short, non-invasive test is a great tool to track patient progress and enhance our understanding of how your brain is functioning.

❖ **RealEyes by Micromedical**: Video recording of eye movements is extremely helpful in treating patients with balance disorders, dizziness, and vertigo. Specific parts of the brain control the movements of the eye. Using RealEyes makes the eye movement much easier to visualize, which in turn helps immensely with determining brain malfunction. Visit www.micromedical.com for more information.

❖ **Computerized Outcomes Assessment Testing**: I like being able to provide graphical proof of how well your treatment has improved your function with research-based, reliable questionnaires. Outcome Assessments are a must when documenting your response to care, for research and other purposes.

I use a five-pronged approach to enable your body to heal your chronic condition. I call it Johnson Neuro-Metabolic Therapy (JNMT). With diet, lifestyle changes, specific nutritional supplementation, gut healing and inflammation quenching and Johnson Brain-Based therapy, I am able to create an individualized plan for your recovery. Several additional procedures help me evaluate other important factors that are often roadblocks to healing. They are often the additional "secret weapons" I employ in my efforts to dig deep to root out hidden causes to your chronic health challenge.

❖ **<u>Nambudripad's Allergy Elimination Techniques</u>**:
NAET uses non-invasive spinal manipulative therapies along with acupressure on specific points in the human body. With NAET I can reduce sensitivities and allergic reactions. "An allergy is a condition of unusual sensitivity of one person to one or more substances, which may be harmless to the majority of other individuals. In the allergic person, the allergic substance, known as an allergen, is viewed by the immune system as a threat to the body's well-being. For our purposes, an allergy is defined in terms of what a substance does to the energy flow in the body. When contact is made with an allergen, it causes blockages in the energy pathways called meridians, or we can say, it disrupts the normal flow of energy through the body's electrical circuits. Meridian energy blockages cause interference in communication between the brain and body via the nervous system. Blocked energy flow is the first step in a chain of events that can develop into an allergic response. Allergies are the result of energy imbalances in the body, leading to a diminished state of health in one or more organ systems."[39]

NAET uses a selective blend of energy balancing, testing and treatment procedures from acupuncture/acupressure, allopathy, chiropractic, nutritional, and kinesiological disciplines of medicine to treat imbalances that lead to allergies or hypersensitivities.

NAET has been found to be very effective for many acute and chronic conditions that are a result of hypersensitivity reactions. Allergies are caused by many things, including foods, drugs, vitamins, chemicals, grasses, flowers, trees, etc. In some people, contact with these substances causes severe reactions.

NAET is an energy balancing technique. It aims to enable energy flow throughout your body, without restrictions. By using NAET, I am able to desensitize a patient to an allergen by applying adequate pressure directly on specific points while the person is in direct contact with the allergen being treated. The process of NAET brings about balance to the nervous system and meridian system. This process is a completely natural way of treating you to help eliminate many of your sensitivities. For more information, see www.NAET.com.

❖ **<u>Nano SRT Wellness System</u>**: A new addition to our treatment approach is Nano SRT(Stress Reduction Therapy). The Nano SRT Wellness System is both an assessment and a therapeutic tool. I can use this system to identify substances causing stress on your body (stressors), and to correct your body's response so that future exposure to those substances no longer causes a stress response.

The Nano SRT is safe and effective for adults and children of all ages. The therapy is non-invasive and painless, and contains no needles, shots, medication, or supplements. This system is based upon Bioelectric Medicine principles that state that all substances, living or otherwise, possess a unique, measurable energetic frequency.

The Nano SRT's FDA-cleared BioFeedback System emits frequencies that are representative of these substances, and records the body's stress responses toward these frequencies. There are over fifty thousand frequencies (stressors) stored in the Nano SRT proprietary database. As baseline parameters have been scientifically established for the response toward each frequency, any reading that falls outside of these parameters indicates that the representative substance may be creating undue stress and possibly contributing toward health issues and symptoms that are currently being experienced.

The Nano SRT System provides the patient and practitioner with a report of findings indicating:

- the substances and groups identified as stressors
- the level of stressor severity for each item
- whether the stressor is chronic or acute in nature

We start the Nano SRT process off with a 100-point wellness system inspection. The inspection takes ten to twelve minutes, and provides me with a report of findings, indicating the items (stressors), in order of severity and identified as acute or chronic problems, that are most likely contributing to a patient's health condition.

The Nano SRT Therapy utilizes the Nano SRT Focus Therapy Tool to transmit a series of frequencies that are developed as a result of the biofeedback test, and which are unique to each individual. These frequencies are transmitted via an LED light to various meridian points on the body. By transferring these frequencies into the body, the Nano SRT therapy recalibrates the body's response, so that future exposure to the corresponding substances now allows the biofeedback measurements (and the body's reactions) to fall within the acceptable parameters. Your body no longer feels overburdened or stressed by the stressors.[40]

❖ **AcuGraph® Digital Meridian Imaging system:** Another very helpful tool I have recently added to my investigative and treatment protocol is the AcuGraph® Digital Meridian Imaging system. This special device melds ancient wisdom with cutting-edge technology. The AcuGraph Digital Meridian Imaging system is a computerized tool used to analyze and document the energetic status of the acupuncture meridians. Perhaps a bit of background will help you understand the value of the Acugragh Digital Meridian Imaging System.

"Traditional Chinese acupuncture has a history of at least 4,000 years. The theoretical construct of this form of health care rests on the idea that a universal energy form, known as chi (pronounced "chee") flows in specific channels throughout the body. These channels are known as acupuncture meridians. There are 12 main paired meridians in the body; "paired" refers to the fact that each meridian is mirrored on opposite sides of the body. The 12 main meridians are named for organs or organ systems, though their energy flow does not necessarily directly affect the organs after which the meridians are named. According to acupuncture theory, all ill health, disease, pathology, etc. are caused by energetic imbalances among these 12 meridians, causing excesses or deficiencies of energy in specific channels.

In the early 1950's Dr. Yoshio Nakatani noted areas of altered electrical conductivity on the skin of patients with various diseases. These areas were found to be points of approximately 1cm diameter, generally in lines following the classical Chinese acupuncture meridians. Because these points offered increased electrical conductance, he named these points, "ryodoraku" (ryo=good, 'do=(electro) conductive, 'raku=line.)

Dr. Nakatani refined his procedures to encompass both diagnosis and treatment. Diagnosis was performed with an electrical instrument measuring electrical conductivity of the skin. By measuring the conductivity of each meridian, energetic excesses and deficiencies could be located. Treatment consisted of stimulating specific acupuncture points to either "tonify" a deficient meridian, or "sedate" an excessive meridian. An additional set of acupuncture points is used to balance meridians that show significant energetic differences between the right and left sides of the body.

Since Dr. Nakatani's original work, a variety of research studies have sought to further the body of knowledge about Ryodoraku diagnosis and treatment and the electrical characteristics of the acupuncture meridians. The results show beyond doubt that the acupuncture meridians are electrically active. Increased conductance and propagation along acupuncture meridians has been measured, and noted to change with acupuncture needle insertion and duration of illness. Further, the meridians have been shown to also conduct light, and produce visible energy signatures on Kirlian photography. Acupuncture points also differ thermally from surrounding skin.

Because Ryodoraku diagnosis consists of measuring skin resistance, much research has focused on the reliability of these measurements. Results have shown that typical skin resistance varies between 500 ohms and 9 megohms, and that acupuncture points and entire meridians can be readily located within 5 mm by measuring skin resistance, which will vary by a factor of 2x-6x from surrounding skin. These measurements have been shown to be reliable across a variety of measurement voltages and procedures.

For many years, these types of examinations were performed clinically with analog "meter" equipment and pen and paper for drawing the resulting graph. This method, though time consuming and cumbersome, was often very effective. Later methods allowed the readings to be manually typed into software programs for basic analysis.

Due to the limitations of then-existing systems and the significant need for an automated measurement system, Miridia Technology Inc. developed AcuGraph Digital Meridian Imaging to apply the power of modern computer analysis to this time-honored method. The result is Ryodoraku analysis that is faster, easier, and more powerful than ever before."[41]

When you have a chronic health challenge, I need to look at all the factors that can have a causative impact in keeping you from healing. I pull out all the stops when it comes to tracking down the reasons why you have not overcome your health challenge. Johnson Neuro-Metabolic Therapy, combined with NAET, the Nano SRT and AcuGraph Digital Meridian Imaging are like having secret weapons to solve your chronic health challenge.

Undoubtedly, as research and clinical experience dictates, I will add to this list of effective tests and treatments in order to provide the best environment to help patients with chronic conditions heal. I truly believe proper testing and careful history taking can reveal your body's life changing secrets for renewed health. I have dedicated my life to this ideal.

Helpful Resources

Note: the capitalizations used in the website addresses below are only used to help with the correct spelling of the website addresses. You can just enter the web addresses without using any of the capital letters.

www.DrKarlJohnson.com
www.HelpMyChronicPain.com
www.NAET.com
www.ShelbyLaserHealth.com
www.WellnessChiro.com

Connect With Dr. Karl R.O.S. Johnson, DC

Blog:

www.HelpMyChronicPain.com/Blog

Facebook:

www.facebook.com/ShelbyChronicConditionDoctor

Twitter:

www.twitter.com/WellnessChiroMI

YouTube Channel:

www.YouTube.com/ChiroNutrition

Notes

(Endnotes)

1   Lisa Girion, Scott Glover and Doug Smith, "Drug deaths now outnumber traffic fatalities in U.S., data show," Los Angeles Times, last modified September 17, 2011, http://articles.latimes.com/2011/sep/17/local/la-me-drugs-epidemic-20110918.

2   Wikipedia® ,"Functional medicine", Wikipedia® last modified on April 25, 2012 http://en.wikipedia.org/wiki/Functional_medicine

3   World Health Organization, *The World Health Report 2000 — Health Systems: Improving Performance.* Geneva: World Health Organization, 2000.

4   E. A. McGlynn, S. M. Asch, J. Adams, et al. "The quality of health care delivered to adults in the United States," *New England Journal of Medicine* 348 (2003): 2635–2645.

5   "Frequently asked questions about NAET," *Nambudripad's Allergy Elimination Techniques,* last modified on April 14, 2012, http://www.naet.com/Patients/faq.aspx#1

6   "What are Nambudripad's Allergy Elimination Techniques?," *Nambudripad's Allergy Elimination Techniques,* last modified on April 14, 2012, http://www.naet.com/Patients/whatsnaet.aspx

7   Please note: The Nano SRT System does not diagnose, treat, cure, or prevent any diseases or conditions.

8   Katie Gazella, "The pain from fibromyalgia is real, researchers say," *UMHS Press Release,* last modified November 28, 2006, http://www.med.umich.edu/opm/newspage/2006/fibromyalgia.htm.

9   Anil Kuchinad, et al., "Accelerated Brain Gray Matter Loss in Fibromyalgia Patients: Premature Aging of the Brain?" *The Journal of Neuroscience* 27, no. 15 (2007): 4004–4007

10 E. Alentorn-Geli, et al., "Six weeks of whole-body vibration exercise improves pain and fatigue in women with fibromyalgia," *The Journal of Alternative and Complementary Medicine* 14, no. 8 (2008): 975–981.

11 Helene M. Langevin "Connective tissue: A body-wide signaling network?" Medical Hypotheses - 2006 (Vol. 66, Issue 6, Pages 1074-1077, DOI: 0.1016/j.mehy.2005.12.032)

12 Linda Morris Brown, "Helicobacter Pylori: Epidemiology and Routes of Transmission," *Epidemiol Rev.* 22, no. 2 (2000): 283–297.

13 "Balance Disorders," *National Institute on Deafness and Other Communication Disorders,* last modified December 2009, http://www.nidcd.nih.gov/health/balance/balance_disorders.asp.

14 Ibid.

15 "Statistics: How many people have vestibular disorders?" *Vestibular Disorders Association,* last modified May 24, 2010, http://vestibular.org/vestibular-disorders/statistics.php.

16 D. A. Froehling, et al., "Benign positional vertigo: incidence and prognosis in a population-based study in Olmsted County, Minnesota," *Mayo Clinic Proceedings* 66, no. 6 (1991): 596–601.

17 K. Mizukoshi, et al., "Epidemiological studies on benign paroxysmal positional vertigo in Japan," *Acta Otolaryngologica* 447 (1988): 67–72.

18 Hesham M. Samy, MD, PhD, "Dizziness, Vertigo, and Imbalance: Vestibular Examination," *Medscape Reference,* last modified January 14, 2010, http://emedicine.medscape.com/article/1159385-overview#aw2aab6b5

19 "Headache," *Minneapolis Clinic of Neurology*, last modified January 1 2010, http://www.minneapolisclinic.com/neurology-topic-library/114-headache.html.

20 Ibid.

21 Ibid.

22 Ibid.

23 Ibid.

24 Ibid.

25 K. O. Bushara, "Neurologic presentation of celiac disease," *Gastroenterology* 4, no. Suppl 1 (2005): S92–97.

26 Datis Kharrazian, DHSc, DC, MS, *Why Do I Still Have Thyroid Symptoms? When My Lab Tests Are Normal*, (New York, Morgan James Publishing, 2010), xi.

27 Datis Kharrazian, "Mastering the Thyroid" (presentation, Santa Monica, CA, September 17–19, 2010).

28 Ibid.

29 Kharrazian, *Why Do I Still Have Thyroid Symptoms*, 81.

30 Kharrazian, "Mastering the Thyroid" (presentation).

31 Kharrazian, *Why Do I Still Have Thyroid Symptoms*, 82.

32 Kharrazian, "Mastering the Thyroid" (presentation).

33 K. Poppe, et al., "The role of thyroid autoimmunity in fertility and pregnancy," *Nature Clinical Practice, Endocrinology & Metabolism* 4, no. 7 (2008): 394–405.

34 Kharrazian, "Mastering the Thyroid" (presentation).

35 Ibid.

36 Ibid.

37 Maes M. Kubera M. Leunis JC, "The gut-brain barrier in major depression: intestinal mucosal dysfunction with an increased translocation of LPS from gram negative enterobacteria (leaky gut) plays a role in the inflammatory pathophysiology of depression," *PubMed Reference*, last modified May 31, 2012, http://www.ncbi.nlm.nih.gov/pubmed/18283240

38 R. Melillo, *Disconnected Kids: the groundbreaking brain balance program for children with autism, ADHD, dyslexia, and other neurological disorders*, (New York: Penguin Group Inc., 2010), 21–22.

39 "Frequently asked questions about NAET," *Nambudripad's Allergy Elimination Techniques*, last modified on April 14, 2012, http://www.naet.com/Patients/faq.aspx#1

40 Please note: The Nano SRT System does not diagnose, treat, cure, or prevent any diseases or conditions.

41 Adrian Larsen, "History of Graphing, " Miridia Acupuncture Technology, Last modified April 30, 2012, http://www.miridiatech.com/products/acugraph/features/history.php

Alphabetical Index

Symptoms Index

Diagnoses Index

Made in the USA
San Bernardino, CA
08 November 2016